Decision Assessment and Counseling in Abortion Care: Philosophy and Practice

Kate –

You will do amazing work – for women and all people – all over this world. Thank you for your dedication to this movement.

Alissa

Decision Assessment and Counseling in Abortion Care: Philosophy and Practice

Alissa C. Perrucci

ROWMAN & LITTLEFIELD PUBLISHERS, INC.
Lanham • Boulder • New York • Toronto • Plymouth, UK

Published in the United States of America
by Rowman & Littlefield Publishers, Inc.
A wholly owned subsidiary of The Rowman & Littlefield Publishing Group, Inc.
4501 Forbes Boulevard, Suite 200, Lanham, Maryland 20706
www.rowmanlittlefield.com

Estover Road
Plymouth PL6 7PY
United Kingdom

British Library Cataloguing in Publication Information Available

Library of Congress Cataloging-in-Publication Data

Perrucci, Alissa C., 1970-
  Decision assessment and counseling in abortion care : philosophy and practice / Alissa
C. Perrucci.
     p. ; cm.
  Includes bibliographical references and index.
  ISBN 978-1-4422-1456-9 (cloth : alk. paper) — ISBN 978-1-4422-1458-3 (electronic)
  I. Title.
  [DNLM: 1. Abortion, Induced—psychology. 2. Abortion Applicants—psychology. 3.
Counseling. 4. Decision Making. 5. Family Planning Services. WQ 440]

  618.29—dc23
                                                                    2011051123

∞™ The paper used in this publication meets the minimum requirements of American
National Standard for Information Sciences—Permanence of Paper for Printed Library
Materials, ANSI/NISO Z39.48-1992.

Printed in the United States of America

To the Counselors

Contents

Foreword   ix

Preface   xiii

Acknowledgments   xvii

Introduction: Transforming the Way We Think about Ourselves
and Our Work   xxi

1   What Is Abortion Counseling?   1

2   The Decision Assessment   19

3   Decision Counseling for Emotional Conflict   27

4   Decision Counseling for Spiritual Conflict   59

5   Decision Counseling for Moral Conflict   87

6   Decision Counseling for Ambivalence   117

7   Understanding Informed Consent   153

8   Decision Counseling for Positive Pregnancy Test Results   173

Bibliography   195

Index   201

About the Author   205

Foreword

Alissa Perrucci and I first met in the year 2001 at the twenty-fourth National Abortion Federation annual conference. At this time the second edition of my book *Abortion & Options Counseling: A Comprehensive Reference* was six years old, which is about the same age as Alissa was when I first became an abortion counselor. When we met, she told me how much she valued and used my book. It always gratifies me to know it is serving its purpose: to help others give compassionate care to women seeking an abortion without as much trial-and-error as I had gone through when starting out in 1976 at the Hope Clinic for Women.

Neither Alissa nor I knew at our first meeting that ten years later she'd be asking me whether I would read a chapter of the book she was writing on abortion counseling and whether I would give her my opinion—was it worth continuing? I had only to read a few pages and shot back my reply: "Hell, yes!" (or something to that effect). I feel like an old pioneer woman when I say, "Back then, we didn't have a book on abortion counseling." We'd do it, learn from each other and from the women we were serving. What we knew for sure was that we were committed to "being there" for women when they needed an abortion. As the years went by, we found out more and more what "being there" meant. For one thing, it meant being "patient centered."

The importance of being patient centered is central in this book. Alissa teaches the reader about patient-centered counseling through her philosophy of abortion counseling and her elegant framework that puts this approach into practice. She introduces her three-step framework early in the book and demonstrates how to use it throughout. She emphasizes active listening, not assuming you and the patient share the same definition of the words she uses, and asking the kinds of questions that will help to understand her meaning and elicit the patient's own answers to her dilemmas.

When reading example after example of how to ask the questions that lead to clarification and understanding, I was reminded of a humbling experience of my own. Once when I was explaining the abortion procedure to an eighteen-year-old who had never had a pelvic exam, she became startled and asked, "Is it a girl or a boy?" It took me a moment to register what I assumed was a sudden change of direction in the conversation, and when I replied, "At this early stage of pregnancy, there's no way of telling, but maybe we can talk about what it might mean to you," she shook her head. Shrinking back in her chair, with eyes wide, she said, "I mean, is the doctor a girl or a guy who's gonna be looking at me down there?"

In each chapter, Alissa makes liberal use of true-to-life dialogues between counselor and patient to illustrate how to use her three-step framework when the woman expresses distress about her moral principles, her feelings, or her spiritual beliefs. The reader is shown how the conversation could proceed when a woman says, "I'm afraid God thinks abortion is a sin," "I'm worried God will punish me," or "I don't believe in abortion, but this is what I have to do!" This book covers some of the most common but profound dilemmas women may reveal to you. Another essential aspect of abortion counseling covered in this book is self-reflection. Alissa leads you through self-awareness exercises to help you clarify your own beliefs and feelings, so when you come face to face with patients' spiritual conundrums, conflicting feelings, and moral dilemmas, you know what's yours and what's hers.

Alissa and I heartily agree that abortion counseling often empowers women by validating and normalizing their decision and feelings in a culture where anti-abortion proponents stigmatize and judge them. In one of the journals we keep in the dressing room at Hope Clinic for women to write in before their procedure, I found this quote from one of our patients: "I entered this clinic a nervous wreck, but I'm going to leave it a strong woman. Thank you!" I have no doubt that Alissa has received similar notes of gratitude from women whose lives she has touched. She has made a major contribution to the field of abortion and options counseling with this book, which I'm sure will become an indispensable addition to abortion care providers' training programs. I certainly will be using it as an integral part of the Hope Clinic for Women's counseling staff training.

Anne Baker, MA
Director of Counseling
The Hope Clinic for Women, Ltd.

Author of *Abortion and Options Counseling: A Comprehensive Reference*, and the booklets *Coping Well After an Abortion, For Men Before and After an Abortion*, and *Spiritual Comfort* (coauthor, Rev. Annie Clark)

Coauthor of the chapter on abortion counseling, education, and informed consent in the medical textbooks *A Clinician's Guide to Medical and Surgical Abortion* (1999) and *Management of Unintended and Abnormal Pregnancy* (2009)
Recipient of the 1993 National Abortion Federation's Lalor Burdick Award
Recipient of the 2010 Faith Aloud's Reproductive Justice Award

Preface

This project began many years ago when my supervisor Debbie Cain taught me her technique of abortion counseling in a freestanding, nonprofit clinic. Debbie taught me how to *be* an abortion counselor, how to think about and evaluate conflict and ambivalence, schooled me in the nuances of decision making, and showed me how to negotiate patients' distress and the distress of their families. She had great faith in my clinical judgment and empowered me to trust my intuitive perceptions and stand behind my conclusions. Even after leaving Debbie's clinic, I wasn't done learning yet. It took many years of thinking, writing, and talking about abortion counseling to be able to conceptualize and document the method that I use today. It is because of Debbie's supervision and guidance that I was inspired to continue working in abortion care, devise my approach and framework for decision counseling, and ultimately write this book. In the abortion care community, there has been a long-standing movement to advance an understanding of the value of abortion counseling. During those days working with Debbie, I was exposed to the teachings of these advocates. Looking back, I can see the expanse of their influence and how it shaped my perspective. I am honored to know and work with many of these women today.

When I began my first job as an abortion counselor, I was desperate to read and learn as much as I could to help me navigate through the complex feelings and life situations that patients brought to the clinic. Anne Baker's *Abortion and Options Counseling: A Comprehensive Reference* was my lifeline. It is an extensive account of the range of scenarios that counselors face in their work, including the most difficult and challenging situations. Debbie had Anne's book on her shelf, and I purchased a copy of my own during my first weeks at the clinic. It was a resource that helped me feel more secure in my work and more confident that I was on the right track. It provided the answer to the ever-present question, "What can I say to help her?" This book is a must-read for every abortion counselor and has served me as an indispensable reference and guide. To this day, I still hear it referred to as the counselors' bible. It most certainly was for me. When I embarked on this project, I sent Anne several chapters to get her feedback. It took all of my courage to do so—without Anne Baker's approval I wasn't sure that I would have had the heart to continue! We scheduled a call to talk about her impressions. Her praise for my writing was so generous; I felt as if I had been handed a torch and encouraged to continue what she and so many others had begun. With her words of support, I returned to my writing with a new sense of purpose and responsibility.

During those early years working with Debbie I also turned to publications intended to help patients though their decision-making journey as teaching tools for counseling. *The Pregnancy Options Workbook*, written by Margaret (Peg) Johnston, helped to orient and develop my thinking. Designed as a guide to help women with pregnancy decision making, this workbook should be considered required reading for counselors as well. It takes patients through a journey to explore their feelings, thoughts, values, and goals in order to clarify their decision-making process. The exercises in the workbook, while designed for patients, inform counselors on how to frame conversations about ambivalence, one of the most difficult counseling skills to master.

Charlotte Taft, director of the Abortion Care Network, and Peg Johnston, founding president of the Abortion Conversation Project, are two key figures who have spoken and written on the role of high-quality abortion counseling in postabortion emotional health for many years. Along with Anne Baker, Terry Beresford, Claire Keyes, and Amy Hagstrom Miller, these women spearheaded the movement to create a dialogue about the moral, ethical, and spiritual aspects of the abortion decision, abortion counseling, and postabortion emotional health. They have spoken and written about the importance of attending to women's emotions in counseling and creating a space for spiritual healing. I was exposed to their philosophies of counseling at national meetings in my early years working at the clinic. The work of each of these women can be found online and at professional conferences. I would encourage readers to link to them through the Abortion Care Network, the Abortion Conversation Project, the Hope Clinic for Women, Allegheny Reproductive Health Center, and Whole Woman's Health websites and learn more about the philosophy and practice behind the movement of high-quality abortion counseling. Their efforts continue to inspire the next generation of abortion counselors; I am indebted to their groundbreaking work.

My approach and framework for counseling also come from my graduate training in clinical psychology. I have been fortunate to have gleaned a wealth of knowledge from supervisors, professors, and mentors over the years, each with a distinct approach to clinical work. I have learned much more from my failures than from my successes. My ability to distill the *what* and the *how* of this philosophy and practice comes from the fact that, for me, learning to do good clinical work was not intuitive or easy. I need to slowly digest material before I can organize my thoughts. I also strive to understand the foundations of concepts before I imagine their practical application. It has taken me a long time to distill the major principles of all the wisdom imparted from my teachers, but I am grateful for the wealth and breadth of guidance and inspiration.

The philosophy that grounds this book is first and foremost *humanistic* and patient centered: what the patient brings to the counseling conversation is central; the patient's feelings and experiences are validated and normalized (Rogers 1951). A space is created for difficult emotions to be expressed. The patient's discourse, or story, guides the conversation. Second, it is *phenomenological* in its style of inquiry; a shared understanding of emotions and experiences is not taken for granted. The patient is considered an expert on her experience, and the counselor's approach is one of curiosity, a desire to learn from the patient, and a willingness to set aside assumptions (Ellenberger 1958). Third, it is *existential* in its reverence for the meaning of abortion as an event in the reproductive life span where issues of human freedom are central (May 1958). It is also sensitive to the burdens of that freedom and the suffering that arises therein. Ultimately, the freedom to make the decision whether or not to continue a pregnancy is a decision that realizes the autonomy, agency, and personhood of women.

The phenomenological approach is well suited as an approach to decision counseling. Phenomenology is a method of exploring, researching, and investigating our world and our experiences within it (Giorgi 1970). It is an empirical (data-driven) method that excels as a means to understanding human experience. It has a structure, protocols, and standards much like any other method of inquiry (Fischer 2006). It is particularly useful in the investigation of experiential or psychological topics because it is qualitative and requires a degree of self-awareness and self-reflection on the part of the investigator (Fischer and Wertz 1979; Walsh 2003). In part, that means that it is a way of understanding phenomena from the ground up—from a foundational level—and giving them a space to be revealed and understood from different levels of depth, breadth, and perspective before any hard and fast conclusions are reached.

This approach is also particularly useful in psychotherapy and counseling psychology (Wertz 2005). When most people seek psychotherapy, they want their therapist to set aside any assumptions before drawing conclusions. We prefer therapists who are astute and attentive listeners and ones who have a heightened awareness of their own values or beliefs and how those affect their interactions with others. Clearly, psychologists and other mental health professionals have their own opinions. In their professional role, however, they are expected to be nonjudgmental, compassionate, and empathetic at the most foundational level. It does not imply a state of having no values, beliefs, or assumptions—quite the opposite. Part of the work of understanding and clarifying phenomena is the expectation that the investigator—be it therapist or researcher—will engage those assumptions throughout the investigatory process and acknowledge how they shift and change. In this same vein, readers of this book are encouraged to pay attention to their participation in the cocreation of meaning and use that awareness to empower patients to resolve conflicts. To accomplish this, we will take time in each chapter to reflect on our own beliefs, values, and assumptions in an effort to expand our minds—and our hearts—so that we can engage more fully with our patients.

All three perspectives—humanistic, phenomenological, and existential—have influenced my belief that women's decision making around pregnancy, and specifically, decision making around abortion, is grounded in the concern for other persons, infused by personal values that support the significance and importance of the commitment to raise children, and reinforced by honor and respect for oneself as a caregiver. These three perspectives challenge us to understand and describe what it means to be human and to acknowledge the strength that is necessary to truly accept both the austerity and ambiguity within which difficult life decisions are often made. With these approaches, one can glimpse the wisdom necessary to bear witness to human suffering, yet trust in human resilience.

Acknowledgments

As with many writing projects, getting started was the biggest hurdle. The catalyst for me was the MeetUp.com writing group *Shut Up and Write!*, created by Rennie Saunders, which I found online and joined. Each Tuesday after work, I met Rennie's group at a café in downtown San Francisco. The dread of writing in isolation began to lift. After composing longhand in a series of notebooks for several months with his group, I was ready to move to a more solitary phase at home on my computer over countless nights after work and on weekends. Sustaining my motivation during this difficult initial time was my coach Lisa Berg. Lisa helped me clarify my goals and find ways to eliminate obstacles; I very much appreciate her constant faith and optimism.

Many of my colleagues at the University of California, San Francisco lent their wisdom and experience in writing and publishing and provided much encouragement. The leadership of Diana Greene Foster and Tracy Weitz at Advancing New Standards in Reproductive Health (ANSIRH) at the Bixby Center for Global Reproductive Health at the University of California, San Francisco helped me maintain focus and purpose; they reminded me how the book would contribute to the body of work on the social and emotional aspects of abortion. Carole Joffe, Lori Freedman, and Katrina Kimport, also at ANSIRH, advised me on critical aspects of the book proposal and tips for finding a publisher, for which I am very appreciative.

I am exceptionally privileged to work with the country's leading experts on abortion provision and training. I am honored to serve alongside these heroes who have dedicated their lives to keeping abortion legal, accessible, safe, and affordable to women who face myriad health, economic, and psychosocial barriers to accessing care. In the clinic where I work, abortion counseling has elevated status. Counselors are permitted to spend time with patients, and the work that we do is considered to be as important as the medical components. It is humbling and exhilarating to receive praise and acknowledgment from the giants in our movement—the faculty in the Department of Obstetrics,Gynecology, & Reproductive Sciences—especially Philip Darney, Uta Landy, and the clinic's extraordinarily dedicated medical director, Eleanor Drey. I feel very fortunate that these colleagues, who have achieved so much in their careers, continually endorse the importance of high-quality abortion counseling. Also, during this time of pairing a challenging job with an all-consuming writing project, my supervisor, Jane Meier, looked out for me and saw that I was recognized for my accomplishments.

I am also fortunate to have many close friends who are my associates in the fields of family planning, abortion, public health, and psychology. Our friendships consist of tight bonds that weave our work and personal lives together; our conversations invariably center on the exchange of impassioned ideas about human rights and reproductive justice. There were many friends who read chapters and provided important feedback that shaped the course of the book: Heather Gould, Kate Cockrill, Lisa Berg, Anne Baker, Tabby Harken, Radha Lewis, Darcy Baxter, Eleanor Drey, and Jenny Severns. I am additionally grateful to my dear friend Parker Dockray, for whose leadership and dedication to this movement I have constant admiration, and whose critical thinking and advice have influenced the way that I think and work in this field. Through this entire endeavor I could not have survived without the support of Jesse Adelman, who has always believed in me and has been my constant sounding board for both my struggles and epiphanies. My parents, Carolyn C. Perrucci and Robert Perrucci, have shaped my perspective on the world and taught me to how to think and how to write. I thank them for the inspiration to create.

This book would not have become what it is today if it were not for the counselors at the Women's Options Center: Ana Mendoza, Christine Locher, Elizabeth Johns, Erin Tolva, Ilana Silverstein, Indiana Saenz, Julie Ramirez, Lauren Quan, Liz Cretti, Luz Betancourt, Maria Steller, Megan Tolva, Selena Phipps, Tatiana Escobar, and Zuleima Aguilar. For the past four years, they have been the recipients of my trainings, readings, flowcharts, and handouts. They endured countless revisions to my explanations and descriptions. They listened attentively and patiently as the material gained clarity, consistency, and focus. With unbounded enthusiasm, they persistently and bravely applied what they learned. Their feedback shaped the course of my thinking. The greatest compliment has been watching them change before my eyes as they became more comfortable, skilled, adventurous, and independent. They have transformed lives.

Finally, I thank the team at Rowman & Littlefield for taking the manuscript into the abortion care community and discovering the need and desire for more contributions to this field. I have great appreciation for the time that Sarah Stanton, Suzanne I. Staszak-Silva, Evan Wiig, and Christopher Basso contributed toward the success of this project.

Introduction

Transforming the Way We Think about Ourselves and Our Work

Two of the most fascinating questions to ask a person who is interested in being a counselor in an abortion clinic are, "What do you believe is the purpose of abortion counseling?" and "What, in your opinion, would be the gold standard of abortion counseling?" What would be *your* answer to these questions? I believe, without reservation, in the importance of high-quality abortion counseling. It is my personal belief that nonjudgmental, compassionate, patient-centered abortion counseling can positively affect how a woman experiences and reflects upon her decision to end or continue her pregnancy. It is an unfortunate truth that while abortion now is the second-most-common surgical procedure performed for women in this country after caesarean delivery, abortion is the most stigmatized. That stigma fuels secrecy and shame and creates an environment where guilt and self-blame can take hold. Because of this stigma and the politicization of abortion, many women are vulnerable to the toxic effects of anti-abortion propaganda in their families and their communities. Furthermore, many women who have abortions consider themselves anti-abortion and are struggling to make sense of the conflict between their beliefs and their behavior as they find themselves choosing abortion to resolve a pregnancy.

In each chapter of this book, I lay out an approach and framework for decision assessment and counseling that are both flexible and methodical. They are flexible in that each teaches tools and skills that are useful across a variety of circumstances. They are methodical in that each contains a series of steps and exercises that can be studied and practiced by the reader. I use the term *approach* when discussing the philosophical stance from which I conduct decision assessment and counseling. This is my state of mind when I meet each new patient and face each new situation. I use the term *framework* to illustrate the steps that I take in working with patients' conflict and ambivalence. The goal of this book is to teach the reader how to develop a state of mind from which to approach decision assessment and counseling and a framework within which to apply specific tools and skills. That way, no matter what the specific content of the conversation with each patient, you'll be motivated to engage in a deeper, more meaningful discussion, unafraid to witness her struggle, and prepared to guide her through her quest to find the answer to her problem.

Despite the complexity and contention that surround the issue of abortion and the myriad opinions about abortion, for some women the decision is rather easy and clear. Even if it is hard, it may still be clear. My approach and framework for decision assessment and counseling allows a space for this and does not try to make every abortion decision and every counseling session fill a greater space than it needs. Instead, it allows the counselor to quickly and easily determine the patients for whom little or no additional conversation is needed. Respectful and compassionate care can proceed from there. It is also true that not every woman is exposed to hurtful and judgmental rhetoric once she has left the clinic. Some women are rooted firmly in a supportive family and community context that believes in the importance of safe, legal, and accessible abortion care. For these women, a positive experience at the clinic simply serves to reinforce those beliefs and see those beliefs put into action. On the other hand, some women who consider themselves pro-choice can have tremendous conflict over their abortion decision. The approach and framework of this book are adaptable to all types of decision conflict, no matter their origin.

A key concept that is of paramount importance to my approach to decision assessment and counseling is what I call *purposeful normalization*. I use the word *purposeful* to emphasize that what we do and say in the clinic *consciously* is not aligned with the status quo about abortion—it is profoundly different. In the clinic, abortion is *considered* in a different way than it is in the everyday world. We are proud of where we work, unashamed to say the word *abortion*, honor and respect our patients, and treat them with the same kindness and courtesy that we would expect seeking any other type of medical care. In our work, we feel rewarded to work alongside colleagues who embody a nonjudgmental, compassionate, empowering stance toward women seeking abortion and strive to provide medically accurate information in a patient-centered manner.

When abortion care becomes normalized, we model how the experience—both for staff and for patients—can be lived as a normal part of women's reproductive health life span. In a purposefully normalizing approach, abortions and abortion work are lived as destigmatized events in women's lives. Staff are encouraged to be proud of their work and mentored to grow and change. Patients are welcomed into the clinic and are *met where they are*. Feelings are permitted and validated. Angry patients are given respect and compassion and an opportunity to let down their guard, yet there is zero tolerance for an unsafe environment for patients and staff. In this approach, we live as if abortion care were completely mainstreamed, routinely available, and non-compartmentalized. This attitudinal and behavioral shift is part and parcel of the teaching of destigmatization.

The work of purposeful normalization on the part of staff starts on the telephone and ends as the patient walks out the front door. Who are the patients who call out for this work? Women who at first could not speak the word *abortion* for fear of being shamed by the receptionist; women who initially frightened staff with their anger because they were so defended against their fear and shame; women burdened by guilt from the judgment of others. When staff greet patients at the door with "Welcome!" or "Good to see you," it is a first step toward removing shame. This welcoming sentiment and attitude of "there's no judgment here" creates a safe space where women are better able to handle the awkwardness of having to sit together in the waiting room and the embarrassment of having to put their legs in stirrups. The joy of our work is when women are walking toward the exit after their abortions, smiling and waving goodbye to the staff, and thanking everyone for their help. We are so fortunate to have jobs where we help people and receive their gratitude.

One of the wonderful aspects of working in an abortion clinic is that in many settings, it is a place where individuals without formal training in counseling or psychology can help women feel more empowered in a healthcare setting. Patients benefit from the styles and approaches of staff who are their peers and bring a social model to a medical context. This book supports the peer counselor and paraprofessional paradigm by providing a framework in which staff can locate themselves and their skill levels and can set goals for personal and professional growth and transformation. One of the goals of this book is to help readers ascertain their comfort with and skills in different levels of counseling. The approach and framework are adapted to the content of each chapter to allow readers to find a space where they are most comfortable, that matches their skill levels, and for which they have supervisory support. Readers are not going to be asked to bite off more than they can chew! Training and education, whether in this book or in your clinic, can help all staff to feel more confident about their work, safer in their roles, and supported by their supervisors.

There are probably as many different approaches to abortion counseling as there are clinics. The job titles of those who perform abortion counseling differ, as does the content of counseling. Some call themselves social work associates, practice assistants, reproductive health specialists, back office staff, or health educators. Some clinics are staffed so that the physician completes all aspects of counseling, including contraception and informed consent. In other clinics, nurses fill the role of clinician and abortion counselor. In others, medical assistants are responsible for a wide variety of both laboratory and counseling tasks, including the completion of health education and consent forms. There also are many clinics that do not consider *any* of their work to be abortion counseling. However, for the purposes of this book, I will use the term *counseling* to include that which takes place while one is listening to and talking with patients during their abortion appointments, whether one's job title is counselor, receptionist, health educator, medical assistant, nurse, or physician. This book is a guide for clarifying, deepening, and expanding the work that we do with patients and with one another in the abortion clinic. No matter your starting point or your opinion on the purpose of abortion counseling, you can find yourself in this book and learn new ways to work with patients.

Working in an abortion clinic, whether as a counselor, receptionist, medical assistant, ultrasonographer, autoclave technician, clinician, or administrator, can be one of the most interesting, rewarding, and life-changing jobs that one can have. The privilege of bearing witness to women's struggles and successes, helping remove any judgment and stigma, and serving and advocating for women offers tremendous personal and professional rewards. In an abortion clinic, the interrelationship of women's life experiences, both positive and negative, often comes into stark relief. Abortion is a life event—sometimes a very prominent one—in which there transpires a sharing of personal information and a revealing of intimate feelings, body parts, and processes with strangers. All of these things concern women's privacy and women's subjectivity—our way of being as *persons*. To be able to create a space in which women move through these experiences *empowered* rather than ashamed honors and affirms women's personhood and creates the possibility for women to have a positive experience even while undergoing a potentially stressful reproductive health event.

Treating women with respect and compassion and normalizing and supporting them despite what others may think about abortion is powerful and transformative. Your approach to your work is a part of these women's experience. Because not every patient is fortunate enough to return to a family, a circle of friends, or a community that is positive and accepting about abortion, the experience that she encounters at your clinic models the type of encounter that she has the *right* to experience. Working in an abortion clinic is a noble profession. The simple yet profound demonstrations of empathy, care, compassion, and respect that take place in the clinic create positive change about how we think and feel about women, abortion, and the value of human life. Any society that truly values children, their well-being, and their optimal development must be a society that insists on a woman's right to legal, accessible abortion.

Chapter One

What Is Abortion Counseling?

What *is* abortion counseling? How the community of abortion providers defines abortion counseling differs from clinic to clinic. Abortion counseling styles exist along a spectrum, including information provision, health education, and emotional support (Upadhyay, Cockrill, and Freedman 2010). Clinics describe a key component of the patient-provider interaction as the task of completing the requirements of informed consent along with attention to the patient's emotional needs (Gould, Perrucci, Barar, and Foster 2011). Informed consent seeks to ensure that the patient understands the nature and purpose of the abortion procedure, its alternatives (continuing the pregnancy and parenting or continuing the pregnancy and adoption), the possible complications, and the likelihood of any of those complications occurring. It also ascertains that the patient is making the decision voluntarily.

The use of the term *counseling* to describe the totality of the interactions that patients have with abortion clinic staff is problematic for some and may fall short of accurately describing its constituent parts. What does abortion counseling comprise? As in other medical contexts, most patients have an expectation that they will receive a certain amount of information from their provider about what a medical procedure entails; the same is true in abortion provision. It is also common for patients to receive information about self-care after a medical procedure and how long it takes to heal. In abortion care, patients receive this information in aftercare or discharge instructions. Many patients are interested in learning about what factors caused the condition for which they are seeking health care, and thus how to prevent it from happening again. In abortion care, this translates into health education about contraception. Unique to abortion care is an emotional component that is complicated by abortion being the most politically and emotionally charged social issue of

1

our time. This aspect of abortion counseling is its most challenging, most disputed, and in my opinion, most interesting, and thus is the focus of this book.

COMPONENTS OF ABORTION COUNSELING

So what are the components of abortion counseling? Abortion counseling is not the same thing as the work conducted in the fields of counseling or clinical psychology, nor is it psychotherapy. Yet decision assessment and counseling share similarities with clinical methods and models such as motivational interviewing (Miller and Rose 2009) and empowerment process (Cattaneo and Chapman 2010). They also place emphasis on techniques that are foundational in psychodynamic psychotherapy, such as an exploration and discussion of the patient's emotions (Shedler 2010) and the building of a collaborative relationship based on rapport and trust (Teyber 1992). However, the differences are more numerous than the similarities. Abortion counseling typically takes place in a single encounter, without plans for future encounters. The purposes of abortion counseling are many, including providing information and reassurance, discussing pros and cons of different forms of contraception, and answering questions. And at its core, abortion counseling upholds and completes the process of informed consent.

Each abortion clinic is unique, and each has its own approach to abortion counseling (Gould, Perrucci, Barar, and Foster 2011). Depending on the clinic, the components of counseling may take place over time during the patient's visit or may be conducted by a number of different staff members. In other clinics, a designated "counselor" may complete *all* components during a designated counseling session. In this chapter, I describe the following components: information about the patient's visit, aftercare or discharge instructions, health education about contraception, and the decision assessment (see figure 1.1). Chapter 2 goes into more depth about the decision assessment. Chapter 7 is devoted to a deeper examination of the process of informed consent.

The order in which these components are conducted depends largely upon the needs of the patient—this is part of what makes counseling patient centered. If a patient begins the counseling session crying, the counselor doesn't start the conversation by talking to her about aftercare—she acknowledges the patient's emotions and gives her a space to talk about them. This is a compassionate approach to relating to another human being as well as part of the patient-centered philosophy: you are going with the flow of the patient. It is essential, however, that all aspects of information provision and decision assessment take place *before* signing of consent forms. The only component

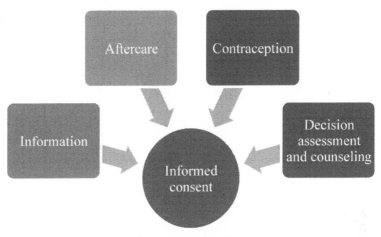

Figure 1.1.   Components of Abortion Counseling

for which the timing of the delivery is flexible is health education about contraception. Generally speaking, a person cannot consent to a procedure if she does not understand what will take place during the procedure, the possible complications and their likelihood of occurrence, or the expectations for her recovery. Consent is not valid until you have ascertained that the patient desires the procedure and is doing so voluntarily. All of these components of counseling are integral parts of the process of informed consent.

Above all, when you begin a counseling session it is important to let each patient know what will take place. I tend to start each encounter by informing the patient of what we will accomplish together. Then I ask whether she has any questions or concerns she would like to bring up before I begin presenting information. I find that most women prefer that I begin the session, knowing that they have carte blanche to ask questions as they come up. Here's an example of a way to begin a counseling session:

Counselor: My name is Alissa, and I'll be doing your paperwork with you today. Together, we'll do five things: first, I'll explain what to expect during your visit. Next, I'll show you how to take care of yourself after your abortion. Then, I'll see if you are interested in getting a birth control method from us. I'll also ask you some medical and personal questions and write some things down on this form. Last, you and I will sign consent forms together. Do you have any questions to start with, or would you prefer that I start by explaining what's going to happen today during your visit?

Here's another variation on how to introduce the counseling session:

Counselor: My name is Chris, and my role is to answer any questions that you might have and provide you with information to make your visit better. Do you have any questions to start with, or would you prefer that I start by explaining what's going to happen today during your visit?

Information and Aftercare

Information about the visit and aftercare instructions involve the imparting of mostly standard facts about what will happen during the clinic visit and how to take care of oneself after an abortion. Both are essential to ensuring that the requirements of informed consent are met. A person cannot adequately consent to a medical procedure unless she understands the nature and purpose of that procedure and how her body will be affected by it. To achieve both of these goals, staff must be able to impart the facts of the medical procedure and aftercare in a way that the patient can understand. The actual information included in these components varies from clinic to clinic because what takes place during the patient's visit is unique to each facility. In terms of describing the procedure, patients have a right to know what is going to happen to them during the visit. As counselor Megan put it, they have the right to know what is going into their bodies (medicines, devices, instruments) and what is coming out (blood samples, cultures, products of conception). This is not a place to be embarrassed or apologetic, but it's also not a place to be gory or use medical language that the patient can't understand. A skilled counselor frames the process of clinic flow and the procedure in a both a truthful and empowering way.

The information provided in these two components should be uniform. Facts are facts. *Abortion Counseling: A Clinician's Guide to Psychology, Legislation, Politics, and Competency* has good examples of patient instructions (Needle and Walker 2008). The patient-centered aspects of these two components come into play when a woman needs a more detailed explanation of aspects of her visit, possibly because the abortion is also going to be her first pelvic exam or she has little understanding of reproductive anatomy. Some clinics save time with these tasks by conducting group counseling or having all patients watch a video that explains the abortion. When providing different types of information, some patients benefit from an approach that utilizes more than one learning modality. For example, when discussing laminaria insertion, many counselors use a dual approach of verbal description along with a demonstration using an anatomical model of the female pelvis to locate the cervix and describe the placement of laminaria. Counselors also show patients sample laminaria and let them touch them. A triage form or a self-report medical history can help staff determine which patients might benefit from additional health education to understand the difference between the cervix and the uterus or how to relax during the insertion of the speculum. Triage forms can also be useful to screen which women may benefit from emotional or decision counseling. An example of a triage form can be found in Anne Baker and Terry Beresford's (2009) chapter in *Management of Abnormal and Unintended Pregnancy* (Paul et al. 2009) and *Abortion Counseling* (Needle and Walker 2008).

The goals of aftercare are to teach the ways to distinguish normal experiences from emergencies and how to prevent and respond to post-abortion complications. A dual-modality learning approach could take the form of verbal instruction while in counseling, a second verbal reminder during post-abortion recovery, and a handout to take home. Another approach would be discussing aftercare in a video that plays in the waiting room and a brochure in patients' to-go bags. Understanding the tasks necessary for optimal self-care after a medical procedure also feed into the ability to make an informed decision. Patients need to know about recovery time, restrictions, and the impact of a procedure on their ability to return to their everyday life *before* they give consent to have that procedure.

Health Education

Health education about contraception is a field of expertise unto itself, and there have been many important and useful writings on this topic (Lethbridge and Hanna 1997). While many of the principles of humanistic, patient-centered abortion counseling are shared with those of patient-centered health education about contraception, this book does not focus on the latter. To be effective and patient centered, contraception health education requires that the counselor be trained in the most up-to-date knowledge about birth control methods, their mechanisms of action, proper use, contraindications, side effects, and protective effects (Hatcher et al. 2007; Speroff and Darney 2005). To achieve competence in describing and explaining all the aspects of birth control methods takes time, practice, and instruction from a clinician with expertise in this field.

Patient-centered contraception health education takes into consideration the patient's lifestyle and fertility goals. It seeks to understand the level of convenience that a patient needs from her method, her tolerance for various side effects, and how important it is to her to not become pregnant again within a specific time frame. It is also important to assess her commitment to using a particular method (Raine et al. 2011) and her desire to avoid pregnancy. It involves the acceptance by abortion providers that some women presenting for an abortion are not interested in obtaining a method from the clinic or may choose one that some think is not "reliable" enough. Thus it must begin with an examination of one's own biases regarding birth control methods and a desire to fill the gaps in one's own knowledge. It also requires enlightenment on the part of the counselor as to how women in different cultures, countries, and socioeconomic groups have historically experienced fertility control. For some groups of women, particularly women of color and low-income women, birth control methods have been promoted coercively. The history of the family planning movement itself is surrounded in controversy around eugenics, and the history of medicine is filled with cases of medical procedures conducted without informed consent. Counselors must educate themselves on this history in order to be able to respect women's elections and refusals of different contraceptive methods. I recommend that readers turn to Dorothy Roberts's *Killing the Black Body* (1997) to learn more about these critical issues.

Decision Assessment and Counseling

Decision assessment and counseling is the least uniform aspect of abortion counseling, partly because it is patient centered and is conducted according to the patient's needs, desires, and requests. It is also the least uniform due to a lack of consensus on the breadth and depth of responsibility that abortion providers have toward working with patients' emotions, as well as lack of agreement on the skills needed to achieve competency. For example, abortion providers do not have a unified approach for working with patients' spiritual or moral conflict with abortion or how to understand the spectrum of experience that lies between decision certainty and decision ambivalence.

The reasons for this are complex. Abortion providers are rightfully concerned about the growing number of state-mandated pre-abortion counseling requirements that serve an anti-abortion agenda over patients' needs and concerns (Richardson and Nash 2006). Introducing more requirements for clinic staff, even if they were motivated by evidence-based practice and concern for patients' emotional well-being, seems overwhelming. In addition, the training and oversight needed to implement and sustain such an initiative would be considerable. The National Abortion Federation, the largest professional organization of abortion providers, has established guidelines surrounding the purpose of abortion counseling and goals for working with patients' emotions (Paul et al. 2009). These standards are critical for setting expectations about what is important to accomplish in conversations with patients. The approach and framework found within this book expound upon these standards and teach the reader how to identify, practice, and implement new skills on the path to competency. Because it is patient centered, it is by definition outside of any specific political agenda. The patient has the answer to her dilemma; the counselor serves as facilitator and guide.

The decision assessment contains three steps: (1) learning about the patient's experience making the decision; (2) checking in about her support system; and (3) planning for post-abortion coping. In addition, counselors may assess for other psychosocial issues that go beyond the abortion decision (see box 1.1). This depends on each organization's values and priorities. Assessments for psychosocial issues can be initiated on a triage form, on a self-report medical screening form, on the appointment line, or through questions during the counseling session. For example, some clinics screen for intimate partner violence. This could be a question on a form or a routine question asked during face-to-face counseling. Some clinics never screen for this issue but instead ask all patients to respond whether or not they are experiencing coercion around the abortion decision.

Box 1.1.   Options for Psychosocial Assessment

1. Intimate partner violence
2. History of sexual abuse or rape
3. Drug and alcohol use
4. Homelessness
5. Depression
6. Risk factors for HIV infection

In summary, the component of abortion counseling that I call decision assessment and counseling can be defined as follows:

The component of abortion counseling called *decision assessment and counseling* is a conversation between a patient and a counselor that has as a central goal the augmentation of the patient's post-abortion emotional health. In this conversation, the patient's experience surrounding her decision, her social support, and her expectations for coping are assessed. Grounding this approach are active listening, validation, normalization, empathy, and compassion. The counselor seeks to understand the personal meanings and origins of the patient's feelings and beliefs. Counselor and patient reframe negative experiences to discover strengths, resources, and wisdom. The counselor offers the patient a view of herself as a good person making a moral decision.

I begin the decision assessment with a single, open-ended question: *what was it like for you to make the decision to have an abortion?* From the patient's response to that open-ended question, the counselor can assess for decision conflict and ambivalence and work with the patient to resolve conflict and/or make a plan for coping. Readers will see that it's fairly easy to become good at asking the questions but that it takes more practice to become comfortable working with all the different responses. For most patients it is a simple, rather brief moment in counseling, yet it is profoundly important. In this critical moment, the counselor and patient's mutual engagement in a patient-centered conversation models an absence of stigma and judgment, communicates the clinic's care and concern for the well-being of its patients, and constitutes abortion as a normal, *moral* event within the reproductive life span.

To make progress toward the goal of augmenting post-abortion emotional health, the decision assessment seeks to uncover decision conflict and ambivalence. Decision conflict typically falls into one of three categories: emotional conflict, spiritual conflict, or moral conflict. The approach and framework outlined in this book is applied to each of these three categories of conflict, along with ambivalence, in four separate chapters. While patients may present with more than one type of conflict, using these categories allows the reader to trace the consistency in approach and framework across varying content. Counselors can converse with patients on the levels of the framework according to their comfort and skills (see box 1.2). They can add levels as they become more comfortable with what they are learning through the exercises in this book. To reinforce the flexibility inherent in the framework, each chapter introduces the levels and then adapts them to each different type of decision conflict using examples of counselor-patient dialogue. Interestingly, the order of the levels does not reflect an order of difficulty. In fact, the most difficult level is probably seeking understanding (level 2), and the level on which most people feel most comfortable is probably reframing (level 3). In some circumstances, such as moral conflict, mastering validation and normalization (level 1) will be the most important. Generally speaking, the levels are meant to be applied in sequential order. When counselors move through the levels in this way, they build rapport and encourage openness to thinking about the abortion in a way that minimizes judgment and stigma.

Box 1.2.   Framework

Level 1: Validate and normalize.
Level 2: Seek understanding.
Level 3: Reframe.

WHY DO DECISION ASSESSMENT AND COUNSELING?

I believe in the importance of high-quality decision assessment and counseling not because I believe that abortion causes psychological disorders, but because I feel that it is an opportunity to transform how women experience themselves and their decision during and after abortion. Centering this belief in the importance of abortion counseling are the findings of the American Psychological Association (APA) Task Force on Mental Health and Abortion (2008), which concluded that women having a single, legal, first-trimester abortion (for an unplanned pregnancy, not for fetal or maternal indications) are not at any greater risk of negative psychological health than women continuing an unplanned pregnancy to term and parenting. Does having an abortion involve feelings? Of course! Women who have abortions are human; they have feelings about all kinds of life experiences, which could include something as ordinary as feeling irritated for having to spend the entire day at the clinic or outraged at having to walk through a sea of anti-abortion picketers. Decision assessment and counseling also create a space to meet the needs of women whose post-abortion emotional health we know less about—women who have multiple abortions and women having second-trimester abortions.

For some people, the decision to have an abortion is a difficult one. For others, it is not. Some women bring a complicated life to their abortion appointment. They bring relationship problems, depression, drug and alcohol use, and intimate partner violence. Having an abortion is not necessarily going to make any of these things better, and it's not necessarily going to make any of them worse. Sometimes an abortion is simply the best decision that a woman can make at a particular time in her life, given her life circumstances. Unfortunately, having an abortion doesn't cure women of all the other things that were going on in their lives before the pregnancy. And unfortunately (or fortunately), having an abortion may be the catalyst that brings to light a whole host of *other* issues in their lives that are now going to *demand* that they be addressed. Sometimes an abortion becomes the life event that helps women to change things for the better. Other times, it becomes the event to which they adhere their life's disappointments because they have nowhere else to put them or no one to help them sort them out, or because this may be the interpretation of abortion provided by their social setting. These are some of the realities of life that make decisions complicated, and it's really important to keep in mind that some appraisals of abortion decisions have to do with the abortion, and some of them don't.

Since the first APA Task Force on Mental Health and Abortion (Adler et al. 1990), psychologists have been uncovering the different factors that contribute to better and worse post-abortion emotional health and coping. An important take-away message from the scientific literature has been that just because abortion doesn't cause widespread, negative psychological harm doesn't mean that we shouldn't be concerned with how to optimize that experience. The same goal applies to carrying pregnancies to term and parenting children. Having children doesn't cause widespread, negative psychological harm either, but that doesn't mean that we shouldn't help women prepare for childbirth and parenthood in a way that optimizes their emotional health and that of their children.

So how do we know that doing decision assessment and counseling is even worthwhile? Several well-designed studies have been conducted to examine the range and severity of women's emotional responses after abortion and whether certain circumstances affect those emotions. When we examine what these studies have found, the results have direct implications for what we assess during decision assessment and counseling. The data point to the circumstances when women may benefit from talking about their decision or when they might need extra support afterward. We can use these findings to inform our practice of decision assessment and counseling.

RESEARCH ON PSYCHOLOGICAL RESPONSE AFTER ABORTION

We know from extant research that there is no empirical evidence to suggest widespread negative psychological outcomes after abortion, either for teenagers or for adult women (Adler et al. 1990; Adler et al. 1992; Major et al. 2009; Major et al. 2000; Pope et. al 2001; Russo and Zierk 1992). A groundbreaking meta-analysis (Adler et al. 1990) reviewed and critiqued studies on adolescents' and adult women's responses to abortion. The authors found that methodologically sound studies provided little evidence to support the hypothesis that abortion was associated with severe negative psychological outcomes or the development of psychological disorders. In this meta-analysis, reviewed studies showed that the abortion experience was more positive when the pregnancy was unintended, when it was not personally meaningful, and when the woman had social support for her decision. The best predictor of depression after an abortion is a history of depression before the abortion (Adler et al. 1992; Major et al. 2000; Russo and Dabul 1997). Also, women who reported greater difficulty in making the decision to have the abortion also reported more negative feelings after abortion (Major and Cozzarelli 1992).

Teens

What do we know about how teenagers cope with an abortion decision? Minor adolescents may be slightly less comfortable with their decision to have an abortion, but one study found no significant differences between minors and adults either pre- or post-abortion on measures of depression, positive emotions, negative emotions, self-esteem, anxiety, stress, and positive states of mind (Pope et al. 2001). These data have been key components of arguments against parental involvement laws, which jeopardize the well-being of minors living in unsafe situations and which lead to limiting abortion access and delaying care (Ellertson 1997). The majority of minors involve a parent in the decision to have an abortion, even when there is no law forcing them to do so, and almost all of them involve at least one adult (Henshaw and Kost 1992). In a survey of minors at family planning clinics in California, a significant proportion of teens planned to use unsafe avenues to end a pregnancy if laws were to change to require them to inform a parent of an abortion decision (Perrucci, Schwartz, and Sigafoos 2007). When minors were asked about their plans if they lost the right to confidential family planning services, between 41 percent and 47 percent said that they would stop coming to the clinic for prescription birth control; only 2 percent to 7 percent would abstain from sexual activity (Jones et al. 2005; Reddy, Fleming, and Swain 2002). Pro-choice policy advocates have used these studies to educate legislators and the public of the purpose of permitting minors to give consent for their own abortions—to ensure that society's most vulnerable youth are able to obtain abortion care instead of being forced to continue a pregnancy and to highlight that the clinic is a safe space where teens can disclose and get help for sexual abuse, rape, and incest. Ideally, parents help their daughters make the decision that is best for them. But what if parents can't? What if a child is a victim of incest? What if a girl's parents are anti-abortion and will force her to continue the pregnancy? What if she will suffer physical abuse upon disclosure that she has had sex? The role of the family planning and abortion clinic is to advocate for teens, follow mandatory reporting requirements, and mobilize resources for girls in unsafe situations. However, some studies have found that younger women had stronger negative experiences of abortion than older women had (Major et al. 2000). It is important to consider the context in which many adolescents make the abortion decision. Their dependence on parents gives them less autonomy than adult women have. They also may present for the abortion as a result of parental pressure, which can have a negative effect on coping (Torres and Forrest 1988).

Social Support and Expectations for Coping

Specific factors have been shown to be associated with better post-abortion coping (see box 1.3). A study of minor adolescents and adult women having first-trimester abortions found that when women expected to cope well, they tended to have a more positive response (Major et al. 1998). In fact, a counseling intervention designed to increased women's expectations that they were able to cope well after the abortion resulted in a lower likelihood of depressed affect after the abortion (Mueller and Major 1989). Post-abortion coping is also augmented when a woman is able to frame her abortion decision and her sense of herself in ways that are more positive and take into account that the abortion decision was the best one given her life circumstances at the time (Trybulski 2006).

Box 1.3.   What Improves Post-abortion Coping?

- Positive framing of the abortion and oneself
- Positive social support and the absence of negative support
- Belief that one has the ability to cope post-abortion

Research has also identified specific factors that can make post-abortion coping harder (see box 1.4). Research on coping after abortion has shown that women benefit from social support when the support is *positive*. Women's perceptions of the quality of social support have been determined to be an important factor in positive post-abortion adjustment. Research on social support and abortion has shown that women who perceive that they have strong positive support from their friends, family, and partners have better post-abortion adjustment by increasing their feelings of self-efficacy, that is, their competence or capacity to achieve goals (Major et al. 1990). In addition, having a negative experience with one's support system upon disclosure of an abortion was more predictive of poor adjustment than was the absence of positive support (Cozzarelli, Sumer, and Major 1998; Major and Cozzarelli 1992; Major et al. 1998). When women fear being stigmatized by others for having an abortion, they tend to keep the abortion a secret; the feelings of stigmatization lead to coping strategies that are associated with less-than-optimal emotional health (Major and Gramzow 1999), such as believing that one is bad or immoral.

Box 1.4.   What Makes Post-abortion Coping Harder?

- Internalizing stigma
- Experiencing anti-abortion picketing and protesting
- Blaming oneself for becoming pregnant

The consequence of negative social support and negative emotions directed toward the self is powerful. Studies on women's reactions to anti-abortion picketing show that negative interactions with protestors, such as being blocked from entering the clinic, are associated with greater negative psychological outcomes after abortion (Cozzarelli and Major 1994; Cozzarelli et al. 2000). Studies on women's attributions for their unintended pregnancy (how much they blamed the pregnancy on themselves, their behavior, their situation, others, or chance) have shown that women who engaged in higher self-character blame had poorer adjustment after abortion than women with lower self-character blame (Mueller and Major 1989).

Overall, research has shown that abortion is not associated with widespread, severe, negative psychological response, either for adolescents or adult women. The best predictor of psychological outcomes after abortion is the psychological profile that a woman brings to the abortion (see box 1.5). It is important to keep in mind that many psychosocial and economic factors that themselves are associated with poorer psychological health also increase a woman's risk of unplanned pregnancy and abortion (Finer and Henshaw 2006). These co-occurring factors make it harder to say that it is the *abortion* that causes negative psychological harm rather than the insidious effects of poverty, childhood physical or sexual abuse, intimate partner violence, and rape (Russo and Denious 1998; Steinberg, Becker, and Henderson 2011; Steinberg and Russo 2008). These factors alone in a person's life history can diminish the capacity to cope with stressful life events. These findings are part of the rationale as to why many clinics screen for sexual assault, rape, and intimate partner violence. The counselor's goal is not only to provide emotional support and resources but also to increase the patient's capacity to cope with any negative feelings that may come up after her abortion, keeping in mind that these may be more connected to past violence and trauma.

**Box 1.5. Which Patients Have
Poorer Post-abortion Emotional Health?**

- Women with a prior history of psychological disorders
- Women with a history of physical abuse or sexual violence
- Women with low self-esteem and little sense of control over their lives

JUNK SCIENCE AND ABORTION

Plenty of anti-abortion propaganda and junk science tries to make a causal link between abortion and psychological disorders. Social scientists who have analyzed the methods and conclusions used in junk science have found poor and biased study designs, inappropriate application of statistical tests, and flawed choice of measures, outcome variables, and inclusion and exclusion criteria (Major et al. 2009). In recent years, we have seen an increase in research conducted by anti-abortion individuals claiming that abortion causes severe negative emotional distress. The design and methods of these studies have been examined by highly respected psychologists, epidemiologists, and demographers and have been found to suffer from serious methodological flaws. In many of these flawed studies, the authors made decisions in their study designs and analyses that influenced results to show that women who had had abortions appeared to fare more poorly. These authors also have repeatedly drawn conclusions from data that are inappropriate given the way the data were collected. In other words, the way that you design a study determines the conclusions that you may draw from it. Over and over, these authors neglected to adhere to scientific principles and overstepped the bounds of scientific integrity.

Even while flawed studies have received extensive criticism within the scientific community, their messages have been taken up by the media and the anti-abortion movement. The tactics that the anti-abortion community uses to dissuade women from having abortions have changed over the years from prioritizing the rights of the fetus to creating the impression that abortion hurts women. The truth, I believe, is that anti-abortion tactics don't dissuade many women from having abortions. Instead, these tactics—forcing patients to view ultrasounds, luring them into crisis pregnancy centers in order to persuade them to continue their pregnancies—increase internalized stigma and shame around the abortion decision. This is not even to mention the ominous and threatening presence of protesters found outside abortion clinics nationwide conducting "sidewalk counseling," harassing women, calling them murderers, and picketing with graphic pictures. It should be obvious that any movement that participates in this form of harassment cares nothing about women. Any movement that uses as its main tactic the shaming, judging, and emotional blackmail of women cannot be considered to be caring and compassionate. Unfortunately, this movement's reach is broad and insidious. That is why I believe that one of the most important aspects of our job is to counteract the damage done by the anti-abortion movement and reinstate a sense of dignity and integrity to all of our patients.

THE APPROACH

Given what scientific research has shown about different circumstances that influence post-abortion coping, we begin to understand the rationale behind decision assessment and counseling. The approach to this work includes both a philosophy and a practice. To be meaningful, everyone's work or vocation must be grounded in that person's values and beliefs. This is true no matter what one's vocation. The word *approach* describes how I have summarized my philosophy about the meaning of the vocation of abortion counselor. It is the sense of purpose that guides, sustains, and renews my commitment to my work. It is also the state of mind or attitude with which one is actively engaged in work. It is carried in one's heart and mind to each new context in which one is called. When thinking about the complex issues that many patients face in making the decision to have an abortion, the job of an abortion counselor can seem daunting. *How will I know what to say?* is a common question. A fundamental principle that grounds this approach is that no matter what the problem, *the patient has the answer.*

The typical stance that we take as professionals is that we have (or quickly need to learn) the right answer in order to solve a problem for a person in need. Many of us are uncomfortable with ambiguity and uncertainty. We want to know exactly how to respond to every utterance and want to learn as soon as possible every technique. We panic when a patient says something that throws us off guard. This is one reason, I believe, why some don't want to ask women how they are feeling about their decision—there is a great deal of fear of discovering the answer! This is completely understandable.

I have good news for the readers of this book. To become a skilled abortion counselor, the first thing you must do is accept that you do *not* have the answer, nor are you obligated to find it for the patient. This may come as a surprise to some and a relief to others. The solution to resolving the patient's conflict—whether it be about God and forgiveness, fear of regret, or how an abortion is going to affect her relationship with her partner—can be found within her own thoughts and feelings and experiences. Your job—and it's a significant one—is to inquire into and witness the feelings and thoughts that surround these points of conflict. Your role is to be the guide. Together you will unpack the moments of conflict and attend to the patient's feelings. You will be able to do this because you are interested in her and her experience. In a good counseling session, the counselor walks with the patient through a tour of an interesting and novel landscape, encouraging curiosity and openness, drawing attention to unusual things, setting aside assumptions, and exploring mysteries. Following this fundamental principle, *the patient has the answer,* are three aspects of our approach to decision assessment and counseling (see box 1.6).

Box 1.6.   Approach

- Listen.
- Do not assume!
- Self-reflect.

Listen

When we are in "professional mode" we may think that we need to be the expert, guide the flow of the conversation, and have all the answers. We get stumped trying to figure out the "right way" to respond. When patients express certain feelings and situations that we find difficult and overwhelming, we panic. When we panic, we stop listening. Then we become confused and paralyzed. In short, this is not an ideal mode in which to have a conversation! Remember that as you begin your conversation with each new patient, you are not responsible for setting the agenda for the conversation. You are there to learn from your patient. To learn, you must listen to what she is saying. Think about what she is *not* saying. Everything you and your patient need in order to have a fruitful conversation is right there. When something she says strikes you and you'd like to know more about it, ask her. Part of the work of decision assessment and counseling is to reflect the patient back to herself and let her witness her own statements. Sometimes just witnessing her story and validating her feelings is all she really needs. Maybe no one has done that for her during this pregnancy. Maybe everyone else has been talking about what *they* want her to do. Your presence as an active, empathetic listener is paramount to removing stigma and shame.

Seek Understanding

Do not assume that you understand what the patient means when she is talking about her experience. We all know what happens when we assume! Instead, inquire . . . investigate. Allow yourself to be interested in her and intrigued by what she brings to the table. When a woman says that she is afraid she is going to regret her abortion, ask her to help you understand what she means by the word *regret*. When we are in "professional mode," we often assume that we know what she means, and then we feel paralyzed and unsure as to how to proceed. If we already know the answer, it leaves us with nowhere to go next. When I was in graduate school, my clinical supervisor, Russ Walsh, used to say that when I was doing psychotherapy I needed to get into the mindset of the detective from the early 1970s television show *Columbo*. Detective Columbo's stance was one of curiosity and openness, naiveté mixed with a heightened awareness of his and others' assumptions. He was humble, and he was never tempted to pose as a professional who knew all the answers. His mantra was, "Listen and look, look and listen."

Self-Reflect

What are the scenarios that you most dread when talking with patients? Is talking about feelings difficult for you? What kinds of situations leave you tongue-tied or speechless? Pay attention to how you react to different situations, different patients, and different abortions. Our cognitive and emotional responses to what a patient brings to the table are the data that we need to help us learn and grow, both as individuals and as abortion counselors. Many of the exercises in the coming chapters ask you to reflect on your thoughts, feelings, and values regarding different situations. Take the time to complete the exercises with honesty and without judgment or self-criticism. Be humble, yet don't self-censor. Humility and openness are prerequisites for genuine learning. Record each exercise in a counseling journal. This will be your space to record the history of your growth and change through this important learning process.

FINAL THOUGHTS

Patience is necessary in order to allow what you have learned to steep; with time, practice, and openness to making mistakes, you will begin to feel more secure about applying what you are learning. Take the time to let the ideas in this book sink in. Practice new skills in small steps. Meet with your coworkers to discuss difficult cases, and be open to hearing how you might have done something differently. Sometimes the most poignant learning experiences come from reflecting on things that *didn't* work and really evaluating the outcomes. This is an adventure that is worth taking. Your efforts to learn and grow will benefit all the women whom you serve. Remember—you are doing some of the most important work in the whole world! Taking the time to help yourself grow and learn is part of taking care of women.

Chapter Two

The Decision Assessment

Most women who arrive for their abortion appointments are sure that abortion is the best decision for them at this time in their lives. If they are really unsure or have decided that they want to continue the pregnancy, they often won't come to their appointment. For some, making an appointment and then "no-showing" is an important part of the decision-making process. Many clinics adapt to this reality by overbooking their appointment schedules. The first time that you talk to a patient who responds to the decision assessment with, "I almost didn't come to my appointment today," you begin to develop an appreciation for the importance of the decision assessment.

The beginning of every decision assessment is the start of a conversational adventure. You're never quite sure what you'll find but look forward to each unique journey. In this chapter, we'll examine the structure and process of the decision assessment in the case of abortion decisions that are made with confidence, are made without coercion, and are supported by others. In the chapters that follow, we'll delve into the philosophy and practice of working with emotional, spiritual, and moral conflict and with ambivalence. The beauty of the decision assessment is that it can be as short or as long as the patient needs it to be. When women are certain about their decision, have good positive support and no negative support, and expect to cope well, the assessment can be the shortest part of counseling and can take place on level 1 the entire time. The decision assessment is meant to screen for problems, not create them. It is patient centered, so in most situations, it is complete when the patient indicates such.

When patients are sure of their decision and do not feel conflicted, you'll primarily use a lot of validation and normalization. That takes place on level 1 (see box 2.1). We typically won't need to seek understanding (level 2) because by definition, the nonconflicted patient doesn't bring up any negative emotions with reference to herself or the abortion. We'll primarily be concerned with taking a moment to validate the patient's certainty or her reasoning for her abortion decision—if she shares it with us—and reassure her that we are here to answer any questions that she might have or address any concerns.

Box 2.1.   Framework

Level 1: Validate and normalize.
Level 2: Seek understanding.
Level 3: Reframe.

Explaining what will take place during the counseling session at the *beginning* of the session goes a long way toward reducing patient anxiety. Women who have been exposed to anti-abortion attitudes and information during the process of finding an abortion provider may be more sensitive and concerned about what the clinic means by *counseling*. Patients may be worried that the counselor is going to try to talk them out of the abortion or make them feel less sure about their decision. Many women who have been exposed to anti-abortion propaganda come to the clinic with terrifying ideas and images of how the abortion is performed. These patients worry that the provider will use knives and hooks to "cut the baby out." They have been told that they will most likely become infertile as a result of having an abortion. They worry that their uterus or vagina won't go back to "normal." The suffering that results from these myths can be lessened with accurate information about what will take place during their visit. That is why it is also so important that counseling include information on how the abortion is performed. I usually ask patients where they acquired the misinformation. After I provide accurate information, I let them know that a major motivation of disseminating this kind of information is to discourage women from having abortions. Destroying myths about abortion is an important part of reducing abortion stigma.

DECISION ASSESSMENT

Learning about Her Experience Making the Decision

The decision assessment contains three steps: (1) learning about the patient's experience making the decision; (2) checking in about her support system;

and (3) planning for post-abortion coping (see box 2.2). The first step begins with an open-ended question: *What was it like for you to make the decision to have an abortion?* When patients first respond to this question, many will state that it was either "easy" or "hard." Sometimes, patients acknowledge their certainty along with a description of what it was like to make the decision: "It was a hard decision, but I'm sure that it's the right one." Sometimes they will say it was easy because they knew what they had to do. They may tell you where they are in life, what is going on with their kids, their finances, or their relationship: "It was easy—there's no way that I can take care of another baby right now."

Box 2.2. The Decision Assessment

Step 1: Learning about her experience making the decision
Step 2: Checking in about support
Step 3: Planning for post-abortion coping

For patients who are certain, it's nice to let them know that you hear them by validating their feelings and recognizing that they have done the work of decision making. In the context of informed consent, patients in these circumstances are providing evidence that they appreciate the consequences of their decision: they have imagined what it would be like to continue the pregnancy, and there's "no way" that it would be a better option. The following dialogue is an example of a patient who is sure about her decision to have an abortion:

Counselor: What was it like for you to make the decision to have an abortion?

Patient: It was easy. I'm not able to care for a child right now.

Counselor: It sounds like you were able to take a look at your life situation and see pretty clearly what was best for you and your family.

Patient: Yes, absolutely.

Counselor: That's wonderful. Good for you.

When you are working on mastering the skills of validation and normalization, you may feel more secure if you begin the practice of learning about the patient's experience making the decision with two *closed-ended* questions. This can be a good place to start; some counselors find that closed-ended questions give them a feeling of being able to steer the conversation to the basic elements of informed consent. Here is an example of how a counselor conducts the first step of the decision assessment using two closed-ended questions:

> *Counselor:* Do you feel certain that having an abortion is the best decision for you right now?
>
> *Patient:* Yes.
>
> *Counselor:* Do you feel like anyone is forcing you to have an abortion?
>
> *Patient:* No, it's my decision.

When the decision assessment yields information that the patient is certain and that she has made the decision voluntarily, the first step of the decision assessment is complete. Next, check in about her support system.

> *Counselor:* Thank you for sharing that with me. Do you feel like people are supporting you in your decision?
>
> *Patient:* Yes.
>
> *Counselor:* Is anyone against you?
>
> *Patient:* No, everyone is being very supportive.
>
> *Counselor:* That's wonderful. Having support for your decision is an important part of good emotional health. We're at the part now where I go over the consent form and then we'll almost be done. Are you ready to do that?
>
> *Patient:* Yes.

As you become more comfortable exploring feelings and beliefs, you can move toward using the open-ended question, "What was it like for you to make the decision to have an abortion?" I'm not a big fan of asking the question, "Why are you having an abortion today?" It puts patients on the defensive. Women's *reasons* for having an abortion naturally emerge from discussions about how they are *feeling* about the decision. I'm more concerned with the *what* and the *how*: *what* it was like to make the decision and *how* they are feeling about it. Fortunately, a great number of patients are sure of their decision and lack emotional, spiritual, or moral conflict with abortion. Many say that their decision was "easy" or "clear" because they knew what they had to do in their current life circumstances. For these patients, I take the time to validate their certainty and then move on to check in about their support system. If their support system is not to their satisfaction, I help them make a plan for coping. Making a plan for coping is akin to aftercare for emotional health. It is important to remember that all we are asking is that the patient be able to state that her decision is the *best* one for her, given her life circumstances. We don't expect 100 percent certainty, and we also don't expect all patients to be happy. We want them to trust themselves and their decisions. We can help them make a plan for coping with the rest.

Checking In about Support

Step two involves checking in about social support. In chapter 1, we looked at the factors associated with good post-abortion coping. Positive support—having at least one supportive person to talk to if feelings come up after the abortion—has an important effect on post-abortion coping.

> *Counselor:* Do you feel like people are supporting you in your decision?
>
> *Patient:* Yeah, I have my mom and my sister.
>
> *Counselor:* Do you feel like you could talk to them afterward if you needed to?
>
> *Patient:* Absolutely.
>
> *Counselor:* Do you feel like anyone is against you?
>
> *Patient:* Nope. I feel like everyone is on my side.

This patient is sure about her decision and has positive support. She has no negative support. There's not much that the counselor needs to do to help her plan for coping because her support system is available as a post-abortion resource. This decision assessment is complete.

For patients who have shared the pregnancy or abortion with no one, it is important to figure out how they feel about that. Remember, your patient is not *required* to tell others (with the exception of minors living in states with parental involvement laws). Everyone lives in different circumstances. What is important is how *she* feels about her circumstances. Can she cope? If she can, then the assessment is complete. If she is concerned about coping, you can help her make a plan. If *you* are concerned about her ability to cope, then it is important to suggest that you make a plan together. For example, patients who have a history of depression, patients who are spiritually or morally conflicted about abortion, or patients who had a hard time after a past abortion can benefit from making a plan for coping. A plan includes offering access to the counselors at your clinic, the phone number of after-abortion talk lines, or the names of local counseling services in case the patient needs to express her feelings after the abortion. A plan also includes commonsense ways to take care of oneself: getting enough sleep, eating right, exercising, talking to friends, and keeping a journal. Patients usually appreciate counselors' efforts to provide after-abortion resources, but sometimes they don't feel like they need them.

Counselor: What was it like to make the decision to have an abortion?

Patient: It was pretty easy. I knew what I had to do.

Counselor: Do you feel like people are supporting you?

Patient: Nobody knows I'm here.

Counselor: How is that for you?

Patient: It's what I need to do.

Counselor: I support you in that. Many women feel like they can't share this with anyone at this time. Would you be interested in the number to an after-abortion talk line? It's a place where women can call to talk about the abortion if they ever need to. It's free and it's confidential.

Patient: No, thanks. I know where to reach you if I ever decide I need the number.

Counselor: Okay; we're here for you if you need us.

Patients are not obligated to take information or referrals. You can offer them, and they can decline. Be sure to support a patient's decision to decline referrals so that she doesn't feel like you're assuming she's going to feel bad after the abortion. While I believe that it is important and considerate to ask women how they are feeling, they have the right to *not* want or need help. This is part of trusting that women know what they need to do to take care of themselves.

The presence of negative support—a friend or family member who is actively against the abortion—can sometimes do more damage than positive support can prevent. Try to understand what is going on around this negative support. Who is it, and what is this person saying? Can your patient avoid this person? The patient with negative support will benefit from your compassion and interest in understanding what it is like for her plus any recommendations for post-abortion talk lines, counseling, and self-care.

Planning for Post-abortion Coping

In the case of a patient who has negative support and is distressed about it or a patient who felt bad after a previous abortion, it's important to assess her expectations for coping. We'll look more closely at other examples in chapter 3 of when it's important to assess expectations for coping. It isn't necessary to assess expectations for coping with every patient. If the decision assessment reveals decision certainty and positive support, it's not always necessary to ask how she expects to feel afterward. In cases of emotional conflict, however, assessing the patient's expectations for coping and making a plan for coping are good ways to wrap up conversations about feelings (level 2). Never assume that the presence of positive support excludes the possibility of negative support. Also, never assume how a patient feels about negative support or her ability to cope with it; ask her to describe her experience:

Counselor: What was it like to make the decision to have an abortion?

Patient: It was easy.

Counselor: Do you feel like people are supporting you?

Patient: Yeah. I have a friend who had an abortion.

Counselor: Do you feel like she is someone you could talk to if you ever wanted to?

Patient: Yeah.

Counselor: Do you feel like anyone is against you having the abortion?

Patient: Pretty much my entire family.

Counselor: What are they saying?

Patient: That I shouldn't kill it. They don't believe in abortion.

Counselor: How has that been for you?

Patient: It's been hard, but I have my own views and I know what I have to do in this situation.

Counselor: I'm really proud of you. Every person has to follow her own beliefs and values. You're not alone. I've talked to other women who do not have the support of their families. Sometimes this can be hard. How do you think it will be when you go home today?

Patient: They'll give me the silent treatment for a while, but then they'll get over it.

Counselor: How do you know that they'll get over it?

Patient: My older sister had an abortion. They did the same thing. It's not like anyone could help me take care of a baby right now.

Counselor: That sounds like they're sharing their beliefs with you in order to make you feel bad but not offering any solutions.

Patient: That's exactly right.

Counselor: Sometimes women like to have a plan just in case they need some emotional support after the abortion. If your family is making you feel bad, you might want to talk to someone who can help you feel better. There's a talk line that you could call to share your feelings. Would you like to take one of their cards?

Patient: I'd like that.

It's almost always powerful and affirming to plant a seed to normalize post-abortion feelings. Patients who often benefit from such affirmations are teenagers, women having their first abortion, or women who have conflict with their decision. The purpose of planting this seed is to prevent the patient from worrying whether her emotional reaction after the abortion is normal. Here's an example of planting a seed:

> I just want you to know that any and all feelings that a woman has after an abortion are normal. That includes feeling relief, feeling sad, and feeling nothing at all. No matter what you are feeling—even if it's nothing—you can be sure that there is another woman out there who is feeling the same thing. If you ever feel like you want to talk about anything, rely on your support people. Let your feelings out.

Once I feel secure about the patient's certainty and support, I will ask her whether she is ready to move on to the next component of counseling. Counselor Chris makes a point of wrapping up the assessment by asking each patient how she can make her day better. What a great example of customer service!

SUMMARY

The decision assessment is often the shortest part of abortion counseling. Describing the clinic visit, explaining aftercare, and selecting a birth control method can take a lot of time, especially if the patient has a lot of questions. Don't feel, like the decision assessment has to take more time than is necessary. The chapters in this book teach a philosophy and practice for working with the scenarios that occur the *least* frequently but are the most challenging. Remember that the discussion that takes place between you and the patient—the words that she uses and the feelings that she shares—will give you the information that you'll need to complete your assessment. The patient has the answer; you are there as her witness, her guide, and her support.

Chapter Three

Decision Counseling
for Emotional Conflict

For each patient whom I counsel, one of my goals is to determine what she needs, if anything, to augment her post-abortion emotional health. My approach and framework are grounded in the research discussed in chapter 1, which concludes that abortion does not cause psychological disorders but that pregnancy decisions can be stressful life events and that there are optimal conditions under which they are made. These conditions include making the decision voluntarily, the presence of positive social support, the absence of negative social support, and a level of certainty around one's decision. In this chapter, we look at examples of working with patients' feelings such as sadness, guilt, and grief as well as regret and selfishness through each of the three levels in our framework. We use our approach to decision counseling as our guide. As we move through different counseling scenarios, I give examples of counseling on each of the three levels in our framework (see box 3.1).

Box 3.1.   Framework

Level 1: Validate and normalize.
Level 2: Seek understanding.
Level 3: Reframe.

With emotional conflict, it becomes readily apparent that the levels do not necessarily reflect an order of difficulty. Most counselors have the hardest time seeking to understand feelings and their origins. It's tempting to skip to reframing, where we can "cheerlead" and build the patient's self-esteem.

However, jumping immediately to reframing can sound hollow and superficial. If you haven't taken the time to really listen and witness the complexity of the patient's situation, she may conclude that she has overwhelmed you. This may, of course, be absolutely true! As you become more comfortable with normalizing and validating, you'll find that your curiosity about what women mean when they say that they feel sad, guilty, or grief stricken will awaken. That's when you'll know that you're ready to move to level 2.

When I come to the part of abortion counseling that involves the decision assessment, I start with an open-ended question. It's a simple and effective way of beginning an assessment of a patient's decision certainty and the voluntariness of her decision. Counselors differ as to when in the session they ask this question. The best stance to take is to be first and foremost patient centered. When a woman is visibly upset, attend to feelings first. This creates a space in which an assessment of her decision will naturally follow. Here's an example of the question that I use for the decision assessment:

What was it like for you to make the decision to have an abortion?

Here's another variation of the same question:

How was it for you to make the decision to have an abortion?

Open-ended questions create a space for the patient to communicate where she is with her decision in terms of her certainty, the voluntariness of her decision, and her feelings, and it opens the door to see what, if anything, she needs from the counseling session in order to better cope during and after the abortion. From this first question, the counselor begins to determine the direction of any conflict that the patient is experiencing. When the patient is resolved, certain, and making the decision voluntarily, it usually becomes readily apparent. No matter how you style the question, it is important that you refer directly to her *decision* to have an *abortion*. If you say, "What was it like to come here today?" your patient may think that you are asking her about her difficulty finding a provider or her experience walking through the protestors. You want to make sure that you are communicating clearly and directly and inquiring about her decision-making process. Let's take a moment to review the three components of our *approach* in the context of counseling for emotional conflict:

1. Listen.
2. Do not assume!
3. Self-reflect.

Be an active, engaged listener. This communicates interest and respect. Be curious about and genuinely concerned with the patient's well-being. If you are bored, afraid, distant, stiff, or judgmental when talking to a patient on the telephone or in person, she will instantly pick up on that and give it right back to you! You reap what you sow: The seeds that you plant in your approach to your patient determine what will grow between you. If you give respect and compassion, usually you will get it back. If you are interested in learning more about her, she will be more willing to share.

Don't assume that you and the patient share the same understanding of feelings and beliefs. Find and follow her feelings; seek to understand them better. Look at the expression on her face. Be aware of her body posture. Listen to the words she uses. What is she communicating? Don't assume that you understand what she means when she expresses a feeling. Ask her to say more about it. Don't assume that you understand the origin of her feelings. Ask her to say where they are coming from.

Finally, self-reflect on what sharing emotions with another person means to you. Before reading on, complete exercise 3.1. The answers to these questions are important and will give you an idea of how likely you are to steer a conversation away from feelings. Months from now, you can revisit these questions to see whether your work as a counselor has changed how you deal with emotions in your own life.

Exercise 3.1

Take out your counseling journal and write your answers to the following questions. Try to be honest and not self-censor. Your responses to these questions will help you understand your strengths and your challenges.

- What is it like for you to talk about your feelings? Are you able to do so with your family or friends?
- How comfortable are you when other people cry? Do you allow yourself to cry? Have you ever cried in front of other people?
- When a friend is sad, how do you respond?
- Have you ever felt guilty before? How did you handle it?
- When someone dies, how comfortable are you in supporting those who are grieving?

Above all, to be an effective abortion counselor you must let go of any and all ideas that you have that a particular pregnancy alternative is better, more logical, makes more sense, or is morally superior than another for your patient. What matters is what the *patient* thinks and feels and what the *patient* is prepared to cope with. Your approach must be grounded in the principle that the patient has the answer. There is no superior insight into her life that *you* have that she needs to discover.

LEVEL 1: VALIDATE AND NORMALIZE

Normalizing feelings that the patient expresses is an important step in letting her know that she is not abnormal or alone. Part of the goal of abortion counseling is to remove the shame, stigma, and judgment that women experience coming from both themselves and others. Stigmatizing abortion is a tactic that is used by anti-abortion groups to steer women away from choosing abortion and make those who have had abortions feel regret. Nobody wants to be a part of a stigmatized group; alienation, aloneness, and isolation are both the tools and consequences of anti-abortion stigma. That anti-abortion groups can perpetuate stigma in the context of the second-most-common surgical procedure in the United States is a frustrating irony and a testament to the power of anti-abortion rhetoric. In abortion counseling, normalization lets a woman know that you recognize that her experience is personally meaningful yet at the same time is likely shared by other women who have had abortions; she is unique, but not alone.

Normalizing empowers women by reducing concerns over their own abnormality, badness, wrongness, or craziness. Normalizing is not something that you'll do only on this level; in fact, it will come in handy a lot at level 2. Once you are exploring feelings, the patient may share a whole host of different emotions that she has not shared with anyone else. It will be important to let her know that you are listening and that she is not the only woman who has expressed these things, no matter how difficult they are. It is important to remember that the purpose of normalizing is to remove the stress of feeling alone but not to take away from the patient's individual experience of her abortion decision. Normalizing is a way to let the patient know that she is in the right place to disclose and explore her feelings, but that you are interested in learning about her unique experience of each particular emotion. It is meant to be a stepping stone to building rapport for further discussion. Here are some examples that illustrate the purposes of normalizing:

Case Example 3.1

Patient: Can I ask you a really strange question?

Counselor: Of course.

Patient: What does the baby look like, after you take it out?

Counselor: Just so you know, that's not a strange question at all.

Patient: Really?

Counselor: Really. Lots of women ask me that. What have you been thinking about that led you to ask me that question?

Here, we can see that the counselor immediately lessens the patient's fears concerning her own abnormality or strangeness. Then she takes the opportunity to use what the patient has brought into the counseling session to explore whether there is some conflict peeking out from behind her request. Anytime someone leads with "Can I ask you a strange question?" create space for her to share what, if anything, was making it hard for her to ask the question in the first place. Here's another example of normalizing statements:

Case Example 3.2

Patient: I'm sorry. I know I must be taking up all of your time.

Counselor: Not at all. That's why I'm here. At this clinic, we believe that counseling is the most important part of your visit.

Patient: You mean other women talk about these kinds of things?

Counselor: They absolutely do. That's why we're here; to give you a space to sort out the things that need to be sorted out.

It is not unusual for patients to apologize for crying, sharing their feelings, and revealing difficult emotions. This is a perfect time to normalize. It is critical that you let the patient know that she is not being a burden to you or to the clinic. In case example 3.2, the counselor communicates that the patient is not a burden, that she is not alone, and that she is in the right place. Granted, really good normalization is also an invitation to talk further about feelings and is going to catapult you to level 2 in a hurry! However, even if you don't feel comfortable delving further into her emotions and want to wrap up this part of the conversation, it is still important to validate her.

During validation we bear witness to another person's feelings, not to certify them as "truth," but rather to acknowledge their lived experience. Validation lets the patient know that you are listening and that you have heard what she is saying. It is a key to diffusing anger and hostility and calming fear and anxiety. This can be challenging because it requires that we sit with the patient and allow her the space and time to feel. People have differing degrees of comfort around emotions like sadness and anger, but as counselors it is imperative that we create a space for sharing them. Making a space sometimes means being silent and allowing the patient to cry.

Case Example 3.3

> *Patient:* [*Crying*] I'm so sorry to be so upset.
>
> *Counselor:* This is the place to let it out and cry. That's why I'm here.
>
> *Patient:* [*Crying harder*]
>
> *Counselor:* I can tell that there is something really going on for you. Take a moment and let some of it out.

Now sit back and give the patient a space to cry. As her crying subsides, reiterate that she is in the right place to let her feelings out.

Exercise 3.2

Identify examples of validation and normalization in the following statements. Keep in mind that some examples contain both.

- I can see that you're sad. It's okay to cry here.
- Give yourself a little bit of a break—a lot of women have trouble remembering to take the Pill.
- I want you to know that it is normal to feel all different kinds of feelings after an abortion. That includes feeling good and feeling nothing at all. There is always someone else out there who is feeling what you are feeling.
- I can see that you are clearly angry and frustrated. I can only imagine what you had to go through to get to our clinic. Let's talk for a moment and try to solve your problem.
- It must have been really difficult for you to attend your church and feel completely ostracized. I want you to know that I've met other women in similar situations.
- You have demonstrated incredible strength, and you are a survivor. I can see how much you have had to struggle to get where you are today.
- It's okay; everyone is nervous.

Validation and normalization are the first two tools to begin practicing. Even though they are the first steps to conducting good decision counseling, it still takes practice for them to feel natural and genuine. Don't be insecure if this is your comfort level; validation and normalization are powerful antidotes to judgment and shame. If you are not yet comfortable talking about feelings on a deeper level, you can offer your patient a referral to an after-abortion talk line or to a counseling center in her hometown:

> *Counselor:* It sounds like even though you're sure that abortion is the best option for you, you still feel really sad about it. I just want you to know that is

completely normal. Sometimes women who come here are sad, and I always offer the phone number to a talk line for after the abortion. The women who work there are very kind and are there to listen. Can I give you that number?

With that statement, you have summarized what you have heard and reported it back to the patient. If you are off the mark, she will let you know—either in a facial expression of confusion or a statement such as, "No, that's not what I meant at all!" If that is the case, you need to ask her to help you understand what is actually going on for her.

When a patient is sure of her decision, is uncoerced, and is comfortable with her social support, the counselor can easily complete the decision assessment using validation and normalization. This also can be achieved using closed-ended questions; chapter 2 provides an example. In sum, a decision assessment conducted on level 1 confirms that the patient is sure that abortion is the best decision and that the decision is voluntary. Any negative emotions that the patient expresses are validated and normalized but not explored any further. The patient's support system is assessed, and she is given a referral to a place where she can talk after the abortion if needed.

LEVEL 2: SEEK UNDERSTANDING

At level 2, the counselor seeks to understand the patient's feelings and beliefs. Feelings can be expressed both corporeally (with her face or body) and verbally (with her words). Again, we start with an open-ended question, "What was it like for you to make the decision to have an abortion?" This open-ended question creates a space for feelings to show themselves. Patients may start to cry. Others become quiet. When a patient expresses an emotion, acknowledge it.

> *Counselor:* I can see that you're sad. It's okay to cry here. This is the right place for you to be right now.

The counselor is interested in learning more about what is going on with the patient and thus gives her a space to talk. Your belief in the importance of giving space for feelings and your curiosity about learning more about your patient grounds your motivation to move to this level.

Case Example 3.4

> *Counselor:* What was it like for you to make the decision to have an abortion?
>
> *Patient:* It was really hard.

Counselor: What made it hard?

Patient: I feel sad.

Counselor: This is a place where it's okay to talk about feelings. Can you say more about the sadness?

In the last line the counselor moves to level 2. "Can you say more about the sadness?" communicates that the counselor is willing and able to bear witness to the patient's feelings and is interested in learning more about them. It is an invitation to leave some of the burden of negative emotions at the clinic. By giving the patient the space to express herself, you are communicating that her feelings are not scary, overwhelming, or unusual and that you can handle it if she shares them. This simple yet powerful gesture can be transformative. As you follow feelings, you join the patient in a very personal conversation. You may be the first and only person with whom the patient has shared her experience.

When someone shares an emotion, there are several ways to respond. Some of these invite the other person to share further, and others close down the conversation. As you explore the potential outcomes of different responses, think about what they reveal about your level of comfort in talking about feelings. When we are in conversation with another person, how we respond to her statements communicates important information about how *we* feel about what she is saying. The same is true in counseling. It is important to think through the connotation of *what* you say and *how* you say it. Thinking about how others might react to your choice of words gives you important information about the implications of your words.

Exercise 3.3

Evaluate six counselor responses to a common patient statement, "I feel sad." Start by thinking about the kind of space that each of these six responses creates between the counselor and the patient. What doors do they open, and what doors do they close within the conversation? In other words, what does each of these responses *allow* in terms of staying with the feelings, and what does each *disallow* or shut down? Also consider which ones are more or less helpful at different times during the counseling session and what changes when they are preceded by normalization and validation. Write your answers to these questions in your counseling journal for each of the six counselor responses before reading on.

Patient: I feel sad.

Counselor Response 1: Maybe you'll feel better if we talk about how to take care of yourself after the abortion.

Counselor Response 2: Is that making you less sure about your decision?

Counselor Response 3: Would you like me to give you a referral for a talk line?

Counselor Response 4: How do you feel about the way people are supporting you?

Counselor Response 5: What kinds of things have you done in the past to help cope with sadness?

Counselor Response 6: Can you say more about that?

Let's evaluate each of the six counselor responses:

Counselor Response 1: Maybe you'll feel better if we talk about how to take care of yourself after the abortion.

What it allows: The counselor is going to provide information on aftercare.
What it disallows: This redirects the conversation away from feelings onto another topic. The counselor is communicating that she is uncomfortable with the patient's expression of emotions. Even if a counselor is staying on level 1, she needs to validate and normalize *before* redirecting the conversation to another topic.

Counselor Response 2: Is that making you less sure about your decision?

What it allows: The counselor can check to see whether the patient is sure about her decision.
What it disallows: Asking this question right after she says she is feeling sad, guilty, or grief stricken can imply that the counselor is uncomfortable with the patient's emotions or that somehow her feelings are not okay to have. When counselors are working on level 1, they need to precede this statement with normalization and validation.

Counselor Response 3: Would you like me to give you a referral for a talk line?

What it allows: The counselor assesses the patient's need for post-abortion resources.
What it disallows: It closes down the space in the here and now to talk about the patient's feelings. When you lead with this response, you are communicating that you would prefer she talk about her emotions with someone else.

Counselor Response 4: How do you feel about the way people are supporting you?

What it allows: The counselor assesses the patient's resources for support after the abortion and screens for the presence of positive support and the absence of negative support.

What it disallows: At this moment, this response may communicate to the patient that the counselor is uncomfortable talking about sadness or that the counselor is not the best person to talk to about these things. However, it is an important question. I ask this question *after* talking with her about her feelings as part of assessing her resources for post-abortion coping.

Counselor Response 5: What kinds of things have you done in the past to help cope with sadness?

What it allows: This is a good question to assess coping skills.

What it disallows: This question could communicate that you are uncomfortable talking about emotions and more comfortable planning for coping post-abortion. It is better to first communicate that there is nothing wrong with feeling sad about having an abortion. Sadness is a healthy and normal response. Keep in mind that it is equally true that *not* feeling sadness is normal and healthy.

Counselor Response 6: Can you say more about that?

What it allows: This question seeks to understand the patient's feelings.

What it disallows: Nothing. The counselor is seeking understanding (level 2) and has communicated her interest in learning more about the patient's experience.

When we ask patients to talk further about their sadness, guilt, and grief, we open the door for them to describe the meaning of their feelings. Patients often simply state that they feel sad, or they express sadness by crying. Never assume that you understand the meaning of a feeling for the patient or its origin. The origins of difficult emotions often have to do with being concerned about the fetus's capacity to feel pain, guilt over killing an innocent life, sorrow over the loss of the pregnancy, disappointment over a partner's response to the pregnancy, or the end of a relationship. Here are some examples of ways to lead the patient toward a deeper discussion:

- Can you say more about that?
- What is (was) that like for you?
- How do you feel about that?
- How's that been for you?
- What's been going on for you?

As a part of the process of seeking understanding of the *meaning* of a feeling for the patient, it is important also to understand its *source* or *origin*. In other words, where is the sadness coming from? To understand the origin, I often need to ask a second question:

- Do you know where your guilt is coming from?
- If you think about this feeling of shame, where does it come from?
- Can you say more about what is driving this feeling of self-hatred?
- When someone says that they feel like a bad person, I want to try to understand more about that. The part of you that feels like a bad person—what is it saying?

When I explore the origin of a feeling, I am trying to find out whether it is coming from beliefs or concerns that could continue to have a negative effect on a patient's emotional well-being after the abortion. I can use what I find to offer a reframing of the way that she thinks about *herself* and the *abortion*. I am also trying to determine whether I could help her feel better by providing accurate medical information about the abortion, fetal pain, or fetal development. Figure 3.1 illustrates the flow of the conversation when seeking to understand feelings.

Exercise 3.4

This exercise asks you to evaluate different counselor responses to three ways that a patient describes the origin of her sadness. Evaluate the different responses to the patient in terms of what they allow and disallow.

Counselor: It's okay to cry here. What's going on for you?

Patient: I feel sad.

Counselor: Do you know where the sadness is coming from?

Patient A: I'm worried that the baby will feel pain.

Patient B: I feel like I'm killing my baby.

Patient C: I will miss the baby after it's gone.

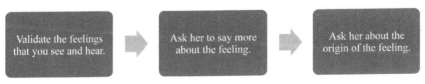

Figure 3.1. Seeking Understanding of Feelings

As you read each of the counselor responses to Patient A, B and C, think about what these responses *allow* or open up and what they *disallow* or shut down. Again, consider which ones are more or less helpful at different times during the counseling session. Also, what does each of these phrases reveal about the comfort level of the counselor?

Patient A: I'm worried that the baby will feel pain.

Counselor Response A1: Did you happen to view an anti-abortion website before coming here?

Counselor Response A2: The best evidence we have from science is that the fetus doesn't have the capacity to feel pain until about twenty-nine weeks.

Counselor Response A3: A lot of women whom I talk to are worried about that. What about that is hard for you?

Let's start by thinking about the space that each of these responses creates for sharing feelings. What does each response *allow* or open up and *disallow* or shut down? What does each response reveal about the comfort level of the counselor? Write your answers to these questions in your counseling journal for each of the three counselor responses before reading on.

Counselor Response A1: Did you happen to view an anti-abortion website before coming here?

What it allows: It can give you an idea of the source of the patient's negative emotions.

What it disallows: At this point in the conversation, the counselor should be interested in learning more about her feelings and concerns and giving her an opportunity to express them. Later on, the counselor could ask about her beliefs about abortion, but preferably with an open-ended question ("What have you thought about abortion in the past?") This closed-ended question directs the conversation away from feelings.

Counselor Response A2: The best evidence that we have from science is that the fetus doesn't have the capacity to feel pain until about twenty-nine weeks.

What it allows: Information on scientific knowledge regarding fetal pain can provide relief for many patients.

What it disallows: While this is usually extremely reassuring, think twice before leading with it. Any kind of statement about concern about the baby, pain, or killing deserves some gentle attention before going into scientific explanations, which can seem cold and uncaring. This response directs the conversation away from feelings. Also, think about what it might mean to a patient if the counselor uses the term *fetus* while the patient continues to use the term *baby*. The patient will probably feel unheard, and it will create distance between the counselor and the patient.

Counselor Response A3: A lot of women whom I talk to are worried about that. What about that is hard for you?

What it allows: This response combines normalizing with seeking understanding of the patient's experience.
What it disallows: Nothing.

Concerns about fetal pain and fetal awareness can be intimidating when counselors don't know how to respond. Patients are sometimes scared to even ask the question, because of a fear that the answer will make them feel worse. The good news is that the current scientific understanding of fetal pain and awareness usually helps patients to feel better (Lee et al. 2005), but be sure that you validate the patient's feelings and give her a space to talk about them *before* you try to reassure her. Concern over fetal pain can be a very intense topic for both counselor and patient (Perrucci 2006). This comes from empathy, compassion, and a desire to prevent suffering. Despite what we know about fetal pain, there is always an aspect that may remain unresolved for the patient. Acknowledge her concern and give her a chance to express what is bothering her. Giving her accurate information about the size and development of the embryo or fetus also can provide tremendous relief. Women may be worried that they are carrying a fully developed fetus that could survive outside of their bodies. Women with concerns about fetal pain may have been exposed to horrible anti-abortion propaganda. Patients presenting for first-trimester abortions are relieved to see the size of the cannula; patients presenting for second-trimester abortions are relieved to know that their cervix needs to be dilated only one to two centimeters to complete the abortion. This information is even more powerful when they have a history of vaginal delivery. It is generally always beneficial to correct misinformation; just be sure that you address the patient's feelings first. Let's look at three different responses to patient B:

Patient B: I feel like I'm killing my baby.

Counselor Response B1: It's not killing a baby—it's technically still a fetus, so you're not killing anything.

Counselor Response B2: Would you like me to explain how pregnancies develop? Sometimes this can help women feel better.

Counselor Response B3: That must make it hard for you to be here. I'd like to understand better what the word *killing* means for you. Can you say more about that?

Let's start by thinking about the space that each of these responses creates for sharing feelings. What does each response *allow*, or open up, and *disallow*, or shut down? What does each response reveal about the comfort level of the counselor? Write your answers to these questions in your counseling journal for each of the three counselor responses before reading on.

Counselor Response B1: It's not killing a baby—it's technically still a fetus, so you're not killing anything.

What it allows: An opportunity for the counselor to express her opinion.

What it disallows: This statement completely disregards the patient's emotional experience and her beliefs. It makes counseling argumentative and combative. The patient will probably shut down after hearing this or at least feel unheard. The counselor's personal beliefs about abortion are not relevant to the patient's personal situation. The purpose of counseling is to discuss the patient's beliefs and how these are affecting her decision and emotional health.

Counselor Response B2: Would you like me to explain how pregnancies develop? Sometimes this can help women feel better.

What it allows: This is an opportunity for the patient to get some relief while giving her control over the direction of the conversation. When phrased as a question, it doesn't feel as much like her feelings are being shut down. Also, this kind of information can give some patients a much-needed reality check.

What it disallows: It's still too soon to transition away from seeking understanding of the patient's experience. Ask her to say more about it before providing information. Think about what you learned in exercise 3.1. Are you uncomfortable talking about feelings? Sometimes we are motivated to move away from emotions to more medical, scientific topics.

Counselor Response B3: That must make it hard for you to be here. I'd like to understand better what the word *killing* means for you. Can you say more about that?

What it allows: This response combines validating with seeking understanding of the patient's experience.

What it disallows: Nothing.

It may be hard for some counselors to use the patient's words. It is important that we become unafraid to do so, especially ones that seem inflammatory or emotionally loaded. A counselor needs to show that she can "go there" with the patient. In chapter 5, we'll explore ways of working with words like *killing* and *murder* in greater depth. Difficult feelings about oneself or about having an abortion are often behind the patient's use of these words. There-fore, always seek to understand their personal meaning. Don't assume that you share an understanding.

> *Counselor:* That must be hard for you. I've talked to other women who said that they felt this way. I want to try to understand your experience better. When you say that it feels like killing, can you say more about that?

A clearer understanding of how she is using the word *killing* can reveal how she feels about herself or about abortion. When an exploration of feel-ings reveals possible moral conflict with abortion ("I think abortion should be illegal") or negative views about the self ("I'm a baby killer"), you'll need to create space for her to share those. Let's look at three different responses to Patient C:

> *Patient C:* I will miss the baby after it's gone.
>
> *Counselor Response C1:* Are you sure that you want to do this? The doctor won't give you an abortion unless you're certain.
>
> *Counselor Response C2:* There's a talk line for women after abortion that is really supportive. Can I give you that number?
>
> *Counselor Response C3:* Other women feel that way, too. Can you say more about your feelings?

Let's start by thinking about the space that each of these responses creates. What does each response *allow* or open up and *disallow* or shut down? What does each response reveal about the comfort level of the counselor? Write your answers to these questions in your counseling journal for each of the three counselor responses before reading on.

> *Counselor Response C1:* Are you sure that you want to do this? The doctor won't give you an abortion unless you're certain.

What it allows: From the first part of the response, the counselor gets an idea of the patient's level of certainty.

What it disallows: While the first part of the response assesses certainty, it's more patient centered to inquire about her emotions *first* and *then* check in to see how she feels about her decision. It seems like the counselor is scolding the patient and warning her to keep quiet if she wants an abortion. The first part of the response could be perceived as compassionate, but that depends upon *how* the counselor says it. Much of what is communicated by what we say is revealed in our tone of voice, facial expression, and motivations.

Counselor Response C2: There's a talk line for women after abortion that is really supportive. Can I give you that number?

What it allows: The counselor is helping the patient plan for post-abortion coping.

What it disallows: While this is an important part of planning for coping, it would be better to lead with a statement that validates the patient and gives her a chance to share more about her feelings. It may have taken a lot of courage for her to share her grief with you, and it is important to let her know that it is okay to have feelings of grief even though she is having an abortion.

Counselor Response C3: Other women feel that way, too. Can you say more about your feelings?

What it allows: This response combines normalizing with seeking understanding of the patient's experience.

What it disallows: Nothing.

This patient is anticipating that she will grieve the loss of the pregnancy. She may feel like a hypocrite because she is having an abortion but will miss being pregnant. Some women's grief comes from losing their emotional connection to the fetus or the loss of the feeling of never being alone. Yet they still want an abortion. It is important that they be able to express these concerns without judgment. After exploring feelings, the counselor can move toward working with the patient to create a plan for coping with her emotions and maintaining a connection with the baby through a ritual or memento—if that's what the patient desires—that is positive and includes forgiveness and acceptance.

Notice that the best responses to the statements made by patients A, B, and C were the most simple and straightforward. Begin by validating the profundity of the patient's statement, recognizing her bravery in sharing with you, and acknowledging her struggle. Let her know that other women say the same things. Follow that with, "How has that been for you?" or "Can you say more about that?" These simple yet profound questions allow for an exploration of feelings in a patient-centered approach. They disallow nothing. It can be scary to take the plunge and ask a patient to "say more" about what she means. But remember that most women appreciate the consideration. Patients A, B, and C are all sharing concerns that may be accompanied by feelings that are overwhelming and intense. They may not have shared them with anyone else before coming to the clinic.

After a while, you may find yourself in a position where there is no more you can do. Your patient might benefit from professional counseling or psychotherapy—something beyond the scope of the clinic. An important skill of a good counselor is realizing when you can do no more. To wrap up, reflect what you have learned and validate what she has shared with you—acknowledge the work that you have done together. It can be validating to the patient when you thank her for sharing.

- You know, I can really tell that this has been a hard decision for you. Thank you for sharing your feelings with me. Is there anything else that I can do to make your visit better?
- You are really brave; I feel honored that you were able to talk about this with me. Are you ready to move to the consent forms?
- I appreciate your honesty. Thank you for being so open. Are you ready for me to give you the aftercare instructions?

When Patients Are Unsure about Their Feelings

Sometimes patients are hesitant to talk about their feelings, and other times they are simply having a hard time putting their feelings into words. When patients have a hard time accessing their emotions but are open to talking further, you can ask them to think about things that have taken place in the past.

- What kinds of things have you been feeling before today?
- What have you been thinking about leading up to today?
- When you've thought about abortion before, what did you think?
- Growing up, what were your family's beliefs about abortion?
- Let's go back to the time when you first found out that you were pregnant. How did you feel?

When a patient is having a hard time talking about how she feels about her current pregnancy decision, you can ask how she felt after a previous abortion. She may reveal that she felt depressed or guilty. This can open up a conversation about how she might feel after this abortion and how to plan for coping. Questions about beliefs about abortion are often particularly useful when talking to patients who express discomfort with abortion but are having difficulty articulating why. Teens, especially younger teens, may never have thought about abortion before and may not know anyone who has had an abortion. In these cases, it is important to plant seeds that normalize abortion within the reproductive life span, specifically how common it is. I remind teens that as they get older, they will likely discover that many of their friends have had abortions, too. Sometimes women have no idea about how they are going to feel, and sometimes they have no desire to tell you. Patients are not obligated to know or share their feelings with you. You are offering a space in which they may share their experiences; they can decide whether and to what degree they wish to join you.

Shame and Guilt

Shame (feeling as if one is a bad person, damaged, or wrong in some way) can be debilitating. It often comes from an old place in our hearts and minds from earlier, negative experiences. Self-hatred and shame are poor coping strategies. Guilt is another emotion that arises from making the decision to have an abortion. Guilt is a negative feeling based upon something that one has *done*, whereas shame is a feeling that one's very *self* is bad or wrong. Shame is a common after having been raped or sexually abused and can re-surface in the context of pregnancy. When a patient expresses shame or guilt, seek to understand what she means:

- Can you say more about that?
- Can you describe the feeling of shame?
- Where do you think the guilt is coming from?

Since guilt concerns something that we have *done* (or will *do*), it can be connected to feeling bad about hurting the fetus/baby, worrying about the fetus's capacity to feel pain, concern over committing a sin or an act that deserves punishment, feeling irresponsible for getting pregnant, having the abortion when her partner wants her to continue the pregnancy, or equating abortion with selfishness. Consider that there are multiple origins of guilt. Where is the guilt coming from?

Patient: I feel like a bad person.

Counselor: That seems like a really strong feeling. Do you know where that is coming from?

No matter what the emotion, ask the patient to say more. Most people feel better simply having had the opportunity to speak honestly about how they feel. Witness her feelings through normalization and validation.

Disappointment

Some patients' feelings center on disappointment with themselves or a disappointing realization about their partner or relationship. Women are disappointed in themselves for not using birth control, for having an affair and getting pregnant, or for having sex with a particular man. Women are disappointed when men abandon the relationship upon discovering the pregnancy or are simply unable or unwilling to offer emotional support during this difficult time. Sometimes women express how they can't believe they are finding themselves in this situation. They also can't believe they are having an abortion—not because they are anti-abortion—but because it was something they never thought they would have to do. Validate the tragedy, the loss, and the disappointment. Normalize not using birth control and remind the patient of the shared responsibility of her partner in preventing pregnancy. Seek understanding of her experience, and give her a space to express herself.

Assessing Expectations for Coping

Whenever you spend a significant amount of time talking with a patient about her feelings, you can close the conversation by assessing her expectations for coping and making a plan for post-abortion coping. Remember that it's okay if the patient expects to have negative emotions post-abortion. The question is whether and how she can cope with them. Take a moment to remind her that all feelings, including relief or having no feelings at all, are normal and acceptable. The key is to determine whether she has the resources to experience them without severe negative consequences to her physical or psychological health. Assessing her expectations for coping can be accomplished by asking, "How do you think you'll feel afterward?" Sometimes patients will declare that they have no idea how they will feel. That's okay as long as it's okay with them. Normalize the range of emotions after abortion so that the patient is prepared for anything that might come up. If your patient expects to feel so bad after the abortion that she is worried she may have thoughts of suicide or has plans to hurt herself, then you'll need to enlist the help of your supervisor or a licensed co-worker immediately. Refer to your clinic's protocol for working with patients who report suicidal ideation.

Making a Plan for Post-abortion Coping

Always validate the healthy coping skills that she has used before and then suggest some new ones. The *Pregnancy Options Workbook* by Margaret R. Johnston has suggestions for coping with negative emotions and making plans for post-abortion coping. *The Healing Choice: Your Guide to Emotional*

Recovery after an Abortion is another great resource to recommend to patients (DePuy and Dovitch 1997). Many helpful essays for patients, including *Coping Well after an Abortion* by Anne Baker, are available at the Hope Clinic for Women website. Remember that getting a good night's sleep, eating well, and exercise are three proven ways to decrease stress and elevate mood. Recommend talk lines such as Backline, Exhale, and Faith Aloud and community mental health centers in the patient's area. Remind her to enlist the support of friends and family if applicable. Give her the readings and the names of websites that have supportive after-abortion information.

Case Example 3.5

Counselor: What was it like to make the decision to have the abortion?

Patient: It was really hard.

Counselor: What made it hard?

Patient: I feel really guilty about doing this.

Counselor: Can you say more about the guilt?

Patient: [*Crying*]. I mean . . . it's a baby. I'm worried that he will feel pain.

Counselor: I can tell that you're really concerned. Tell me more about what is worrying you.

Patient: [*Crying*]. Before my boyfriend left me and hooked up with someone else I was going to keep it. But now I'm alone. I don't have a job and I've got no family nearby to help me. I got attached to the baby. I felt him kick. How can I do this to him? I'm sorry!

Counselor: I can see how sad you are. You're in the right place . . . let it out . . . it's okay to cry here.

Patient: [*Still crying*] I will miss him so much!

Counselor: I know you will . . . let your feelings out.

Many patients feel tremendous relief after sharing their feelings with an empathetic, supportive listener. If you can get to this point, you've done a significant service for a fellow human being. When you witness profound sadness, plan to spend some time in silence allowing your patient to express herself. As her crying subsides, acknowledge her strength. Afterward, you may want to assess the patient's certainty. Other times, you may feel that this step is unnecessary. Nevertheless, it's always nice to close conversations about feelings by thanking the patient for sharing and for her honesty. You can also remind her as to why you engaged her in this conversation.

Counselor: Thank you for sharing your feelings and for your honesty. It can be hard to talk about these things.

Patient: It's hard, but I feel better.

Counselor: Do you feel that abortion is the best decision for you at this time in your life?

Patient: Yeah, I do.

Counselor: I want you to know that it is normal to be sure about your decision and at the same time feel sadness and guilt. Those two things can coexist. Having those feelings doesn't mean that you are making the wrong decision.

Patient: Thank you.

Counselor: How do you think you'll feel after the abortion?

Patient: I'll still think about it.

Counselor: That's completely normal. When women are sad, I always encourage them to share their feelings. If you have sadness or other feelings after the abortion, what can you do to cope with them?

Patient: I can talk to my sister. She's the one person who knows that I'm here.

Counselor: I think that sounds like a good plan. What else do you do to relieve stress?

Patient: I have a dog that I take on long walks in the park.

Counselor: That's excellent. I'm also thinking about giving you the number to an after-abortion talk line. It is free, and the women who work there are very compassionate. They are there to listen without judgment. Can I give you one of their cards?

Patient: Sure.

After you have given her the space to share emotions, you are ready to reframe (level 3). Reframing offers different ways for the patient to think about herself and her decision that affirm the caring, loving person that she is. If you are not ready to reframe, you can close the decision assessment by acknowledging the work that you've done together and transition to the next component of counseling. Of course, if the patient has revealed that she is unsure about her decision, you'll want to get an idea of how unsure she is. Your conversation may have uncovered ambivalence; we'll talk about that in chapter 6. If she is being coerced, you'll need to let her know that no one can force her to have an abortion; we'll talk more about that in chapter 7.

LEVEL 3: REFRAME

In reframing, the counselor uses the patient's reasons for the abortion—the things going on in her life that make abortion the best decision—as the basis for reframing the way that she thinks about herself and her decision. Counselor Julie likes to think about the patient's life situation as the "ingredients" that you use to reframe. When you ask the question, "What was it like for you to make the decision to have an abortion?" many patients say that it was "hard." When you ask, "What made it hard?" the patient will share her feelings plus what is going on in her life that made abortion the best decision. She may be caring for other children or not be ready to have her first child. She may have health problems; her children may have health problems. She may be in school or have recently lost her job. She may have just started a new job because her youngest is finally in school. She may be struggling to recover from addiction to drugs or alcohol. Her partner may be abusive, unsupportive, or absent; he may have abandoned her once he found out she was pregnant. There are many, many reasons why abortion becomes the decision that a woman needs to make. Once you understand your patient's circumstances, you can help her to see herself as a good person making a moral decision. You can help her see abortion as caring, loving, merciful, and compassionate. You can help her see that it is a decision made out of her values of caring for others and a lessening of suffering.

Reframing also serves to counter myths and stereotypes about abortion and women who have abortions. Collaboratively reframing negative and disempowering ways of thinking about oneself and one's abortion is a way to discover strengths, resources, and wisdom. Part of the motivation behind reframing are the hopes of transforming negative self-directed emotions into a more positive, empowering vision of oneself and one's abortion decision and planting a seed for healing. It is a way of showing the patient how she can think about herself and her abortion in a different way as well as an inoculation against anti-abortion rhetoric.

Earlier I mentioned how the numerical order of the levels was not reflective of degrees of difficulty. In the case of emotional conflict, it is particularly important that a counselor spend time listening to the patient's story and asking her to say more about her feelings before attempting a reframing. Telling a patient that she is strong and that her decision is moral and caring as soon as she starts crying is premature and can sound superficial. Validate, and then ask her to say more. Find out where her feelings are coming from. Once you have spent some time listening and talking about her emotions, you can gently introduce a new way for her to think about her decision.

Case Example 3.6

Counselor: I'm going to be your counselor and help you with your paperwork. How are you doing today?

Patient: Not so good.

Counselor: You seem a little sad. What's going on for you?

Patient: [*Tears well up*] I'm not happy about having to do this. I had no idea I was this pregnant. I've had regular periods each month. I was in complete shock when I went to the clinic near my hometown and they told me how far along I was. They weren't able to help me. I feel movement. It just started this week. I have to have an abortion—there is no way that I can take care of another child—I have three children with my husband and we are also raising three kids from my husband's first marriage.

Counselor: It sounds like you have a lot going on, both with your family and with your feelings.

Patient: I'm so busy, and I take care of so many people. I take care of my own mother and my mother-in-law. There's really no one else besides me who checks on them and makes sure that they're eating and the houses are clean. I had an abortion before, but I wasn't this far along. It's the movement that I've been feeling . . . it's really getting to me.

Counselor: I want you to know that other women struggle with feeling movement. It can be very difficult. Tell me, what is it about the movement that's getting to you?

Patient: [*Crying*] It makes me feel guilty.

Counselor: Go ahead . . . let your tears out. Can you say more about the guilt?

Patient: I feel selfish because I know how much I want a break from my children being so young and dependent on me. In a few years, the youngest will be in school.

Counselor: That'll make a tremendous difference in your life, I'm sure.

Patient: Yes, it'll change a lot for us. I'll still be caring for a lot of other people, but at least my kids will be in school. Don't get me wrong—I love taking care of other people. I get a lot out of it. It's part of who I am. I just feel selfish because I don't want to start over right now. I've gotten to a place where I'm working again. I get up at 5:00 a.m. to get everyone off to school and then drop my youngest off at my mother's house before I go to work. I have to juggle all these schedules. Sometimes I even run errands on my lunch hour to save time.

Counselor: It sounds like you have a system that's difficult and takes a lot out of you, but it works. You've made a schedule for your family that is working well.

Patient: Yes, exactly.

Counselor: You know, I think it is interesting that you use the word *selfish*. As someone looking in from the outside, I don't see very much that is selfish! I see someone who is masterfully juggling multiple schedules with limited time to care for and do things for a lot of other people. To me, that sounds like the opposite of selfish. It sounds like you are committed to the care of others.

Patient: [*Crying*] I am.

Counselor: Your family needs you to be there for them and to be healthy, happy, and strong. In a way, you are making this decision so that you can continue to be there for them in the way that you feel is important. That really reflects how much of a caring person you are. It's also okay for you to care for yourself for your own sake. You are an important person in this world, and you have the right to be healthy, happy, and strong. How does that feel to you?

Patient: It feels right. I want to think about it *that* way. Thank you so much.

In the transition from seeking understanding to reframing, the counselor reflects the patient's life circumstances and the patient's *own reasons* for having an abortion to offer a different way to think about herself and the abortion. The counselor learned about the patient's life circumstances by simply asking her to say more about her feelings. She then listened while the patient talked about everything that was going on for her; she validated the complexity of the patient's life situation. She then used what she had learned to offer the patient a new way to think about herself and the abortion.

Reframing Selfishness

I've learned a lot about selfishness from listening to women's experiences. I always start by seeking to understand what the patient means when she says she feels selfish. Then I reframe selfishness as care. I've heard people say they feel that having children is selfish, and I've heard others say that having an abortion is selfish. People judge child-free women for living selfishly as well as women who have six children and are pregnant with their seventh. People are very quick to judge others' reproductive decisions as selfish, especially when those decisions are contrary to their own beliefs about who should be allowed to have children and how many.

It is very rewarding when you can offer a reframing of the decision to have an abortion as one based on care. Many women are trying to raise the kids that they already have, and others want to be able to plan for their first child to come into the world at the right time. If a woman is not ready to have her first child or her next child, or *ever* to have a child, that means that she has looked at her life and determined that it is not the right time or place for that to happen. It may be that her partner is not the right partner—he could be abusive, or he could have abandoned her. She could be unemployed, underemployed, or in school. Her perspective on child rearing is based on her values—her *family values*—about when and *whether* to bring a child into to the world with an optimal chance for a healthy, happy life. I sometimes remind patients that if they are not physically or mentally healthy, they will be unable to care for all the people who are counting on them. If a woman is having a hard time physically (or psychologically) with the pregnancy, or if she had a difficult pregnancy in the past, then the pregnancy itself can put her ability to care for others at risk.

It is also true that it is *moral* to focus on one's own desires around having children (or not having children) and make pregnancy decisions based on those desires. If women are to be considered fully human, then they are more than vessels for developing life. The woman—the born person—is the moral agent (Petchesky 1998). Otherwise, she is merely property of the state or property of another person. This is the essence of women's full emancipation as human beings. I have emphasized to women that it is okay to listen to what their heart is telling them about which decision is best for them. It is permissible to trust those thoughts and feelings. I usually encourage them to listen to an inner voice and set aside what others are telling them to do. When women make decisions based on their own desires, they may feel guilty. Encourage your patient to give voice to the guilt. Sometimes it is representative of her upbringing—she was told not to put herself first, that women exist primarily for the desires and needs of others and that their purpose in life is to play a supportive role.

Emotional resolution means that a woman has resolved conflicting or negative feelings about the abortion. It also may mean that she is expressing positive ones. It is also entirely acceptable if she *never* had conflict about having an abortion. Neither emotional stance—resolved or conflicted—is morally superior. Women who feel *nothing* about having an abortion or who are relieved, happy, or confident are morally equivalent to women who are not. A patient's stance reflects where she is in the process of decision making and is relevant to the psychological nuances that make up the complexity of each person's life situation. The counselor's job is to work with what each patient brings to the clinic, listen, validate, and normalize her experience, and plant a seed for positive coping.

Reframing Regret

Another complex emotion is regret. Some women have a fear of regret, and some women come to the clinic wanting an abortion but paralyzed with regret from a prior abortion. Never assume that you understand what a patient means when she uses the word *regret*. Ask her to say more about it. A lot of women who say that they are going to regret having an abortion actually mean that they regret having gotten pregnant in the first place. They regret being "careless" or "irresponsible" with contraception. They regret having sex with a particular man. They regret having to be in the situation where they are choosing between two undesirable options. They may also say that they are afraid that they would regret continuing the pregnancy. It is important to determine what the patient means by *regret*.

On an existential level, regret is something that exists by virtue of free will and is part and parcel of the process of decision making. If we were unable to make decisions and weigh options, we would have a different experience of regret. Even though many women do not feel that they have a *choice* when it comes to pregnancy decisions, they are still moral agents choosing between alternatives. The concept of freedom is, of course, different in cases where girls and women are coerced or forced to have sex or an abortion. It also takes on a different meaning in cases where women have so few resources that their avenues of decision making are constrained.

It is essential to help the patient parse out whether she is worried about wondering "What if?" or whether she is genuinely concerned that she will wish that she could *undo* the abortion after it is over. During the course of everyone's life, each of us is going to have to make difficult decisions for which there may be no easy answer. We must take responsibility for our past decisions, see them in the context in which they were made, forgive ourselves, make a plan to do differently next time, and then *move on*. Perseverance about or rumination over a past decision leads to stagnation and paralysis. One's psychological life is unable to move forward. Thinking about "what might have been" or wondering, "What if I had continued the pregnancy?" is completely normal, even when we feel certain about a decision. That's not the same thing as regretting that you had the abortion and wishing that you could go back and make a different decision. Thinking about regret as a normal part of decision making may come as a relief to patients who are stuck in the throes of ambivalence and who are trying to make a decision between two (or three) alternatives. The patient also must consider whether other options would free her from regret or whether they might come with regret of their own.

Sometimes a patient will reveal that she has tremendous regret over a past abortion. One of my goals is to have the patient reiterate her reasons for the abortion and acknowledge that she did the best that she could, given her circumstances. Second, I let her know that she is not being fair to herself. It's tempting to look back on a decision critically once you have come to a new place in your life where it might be possible to make a different decision.

Looking back on one's past with the knowledge of one's present isn't fair. The future provides the wisdom and perspective of having moved through and survived the event in question. It's also not realistic—five years from now life will be different, and part of what will make life different are the decisions that were made in the past. Therefore, looking back and saying, "I should have continued the pregnancy because everything is great now," is pretending that one's life would have been exactly the same if one had continued the pregnancy and had been parenting all along.

Mini Reframes

Sometimes our patients share with us very personal and very difficult feelings. As a counselor, your work stands in opposition to the debilitating shame, stigma, and negative judgment that surrounds abortion. You can give a beautiful gift to another human being by framing her very being in a positive light. Such statements can be transformative and are a way of authentically punctuating personal and meaningful interactions that occur during a counseling session:

- What you are sharing with me is very intense, and I am honored to be present with you in this experience.
- You are really brave.
- You are a good person.
- I'm really proud of you.

Conversational Flow

Let's review the conversational flow for working with emotional conflict (see figure 3.2). Feelings may arise during the decision assessment or may arise spontaneously at any point during the clinic visit. Sometimes we come upon a patient who has been waiting in the exam room. She looks afraid or may be crying. Begin by validating and normalizing.

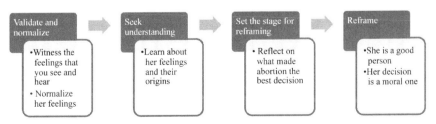

Figure 3.2.   Decision Counseling for Emotional Conflict

Counselor: I can see that you're sad. Go ahead; it's okay to cry here.

Next, the counselor enters the process of seeking to understand the patient's feelings. Ask the patient to say more about her feelings so that you can learn about their personal meaning. Don't assume that you know what she means when she says she feels guilty; ask her to say more.

Counselor: Can you say more about what you're feeling?

You can also ask her to say more about where the feeling is coming from.

Counselor: Where is that feeling coming from?

At this point, the patient has shared with you the negative feelings she has about herself and her decision to have an abortion. Here are some examples of what patients say once they are in touch with difficult emotions:

• The baby is innocent; how can I do this?
• I feel like I'm taking a life.
• I feel like a bad person.
• What I'm doing is so cruel!
• I'm being so selfish.

Upon hearing any of these statements, continue to seek understanding. Remember that you are not supposed to come up with an answer for the patient; you are there as her witness and her guide. Once you let go of the idea that you have to solve her problem, you will be able to relax. Once you relax, you'll find yourself more open, curious, and interested in learning about her experience. After the patient has expressed the difficult feelings that she has about herself and her decision, let her know that you are with her and that you recognize the magnitude of what she has shared with you. You can do this with words that validate her experience. Sometimes, a touch on the shoulder is appropriate. When a woman is grieving and crying, comfort her as you would comfort any other person who is feeling sorrow, grief, or distress:

• It's okay; let it out.
• I know; you're really hurting right now.
• I want you to know that I'm here for you.

When the patient has stopped crying or when there is a pause in the conversation, acknowledge the reality of the circumstances in which she made the decision to have an abortion. If you have been talking to her for some time, you may already know why she feels abortion is best. If you do not yet know her circumstances, here are a few ways to inquire:

• I can tell that it was really hard for you to make this decision. Tell me, what is going on in your life that brought you here?
• When someone is as sad as you are, I know that it was a tough decision. How did you realize that this was the way that you had to go?
• Knowing that abortion is a decision that you need to make doesn't always mean that it is going to be an easy one. It's hard for a lot of people. What made abortion the decision that you needed to make?

From these questions, the patient will share the reality of her circumstances. After learning about her reality, it's your turn to offer a reframe that the decision to have an abortion, given her life circumstances, is a *moral* one. In other words, it's about being just and fair because she can't take care of a child right now or because the children she already has need her. It's about compassion and mercy because it would prevent the suffering of a baby with a fetal diagnosis. It's about caring and loving children because she isn't able to provide what a child needs at this time in her life. It's about reducing the suffering of everyone involved because her illness or disability makes it hard for her to take care of others. Above all, when a woman considers abortion, it shows that she cares about the well-being of children because she takes seriously what children need and deserve in order to thrive. When you are in circumstances where you are unable to spend lots of time with a patient, here's another transitional statement you can make once the patient has shared her feelings:

> *Counselor:* I've been working here for some time, and I've learned a lot about the reasons why women have abortions. Women have abortions for two main reasons: to be able to care for the children they already have and to be able to plan their lives so that they can care for the children they may have in the future. There are also women who know that they never want to have children. So I can imagine that you are a good person trying to do the right thing based on what is going on in your life right now.

With this statement, you are letting her know that you imagine that her situation is similar to one of those stated above. If you've hit the nail on the head, she'll give you feedback by nodding or responding in the affirmative. After you learn what made abortion the best decision, you can transition smoothly into a reframe that offers her a view of herself as a good person making a moral decision:

• I see a person who cares for a lot of other people in this world who is trying to make it so that she can continue to do so.

- There are a lot of people who rely on you. You have a young child right now who needs you to be there for her. This is about what is fair and just.
- I see someone who is trying to take care of her family.
- Your decision will reduce the suffering of everyone involved. At this clinic, we see that as a moral decision.
- What I hear is that you are making this decision because you care about the well-being of children. You are following your family values. When you have everything in place to be able to care for a child, you'll know that you're ready.
- Based on what you are saying, I can tell that for you having an abortion doesn't mean that you don't have love for this baby. I hear how much you care about what is good for children. I wonder whether you could see yourself as a good person making a moral decision.

The different aspects of abortion as a moral decision (as one based on care, love, compassion, mercy, justice, and fairness) can be used interchangeably with different life circumstances. Once you have examined your own values and why you work in abortion care, it is likely that you will find that you have always thought about abortion as a moral decision. Be proud of this discovery and share it with your patients. The weight that you release from their hearts and their spirits will be tremendous, and you will have made a difference in the world.

Closing the Decision Assessment

After a conversation about emotional conflict it is sometimes good to close the assessment with a check-in to see how the patient is doing, especially in instances where the patient was very conflicted and you spent a long time talking about her feelings. At this point, I may decide to use closed-ended questions instead of open-ended questions:

Counselor: We've being talking for a while and I just wanted to check in with you about how you're feeling about your decision to have the abortion. Do you feel sure that abortion is the best decision for you at this time?

Patient: Yes, I do.

If your patient has already stated that she was sure about her decision, then you may feel that you don't have to reassess for certainty. Nevertheless, it's always nice to check in after a conversation about feelings or beliefs. Thank your patient for sharing, and thank her for her honesty. Ask her whether anything has changed. That is a way for you to get feedback about how you are doing and whether you are meeting her needs.

Counselor: Thank you for being so honest with me about your feelings. How are you doing right now?

Patient: I feel a lot better.

Counselor: That's wonderful. Are you ready for me to give you some information about your visit and some aftercare instructions?

Patient: Yes, I'm ready.

FINAL THOUGHTS

The skills that you practice and develop in this chapter create the foundation for your work in the two remaining spheres of conflict: spiritual and moral. They also are the groundwork for skillfully conducting counseling for ambivalence. You will use validation and normalization no matter the subject of your conversation; these are the two primary weapons in your arsenal against shame, stigma, and judgment. Going forward, you will need to hone the skill of seeking to understand your patient's feelings and beliefs—don't assume; ask her to say more about what she means. Working skillfully with spiritual and moral conflict demands that you make no assumptions; uncovering the personal meaning of the patient's beliefs will be paramount.

Reframing is a skill that you will use with spiritual and moral conflict as well, although you may come to find that a lot of the reframing of spiritual conflict involves reflecting back the patient's beliefs and is less a new way to think about abortion. Interestingly, the reframing that you'll use with moral conflict is very similar to the reframing in this chapter, but getting there can be more difficult. You'll need to hone your skills of validating and normalizing to build rapport with patients who are angry and defensive. Throughout the rest of the book, you will use everything that you've learned in this chapter. Allow yourself time to practice what you've learned before jumping into the other chapters. You'll always be working with feelings, even when you find yourself navigating the waters of spirituality, religious belief, ambivalence, or anti-abortion sentiment. That is why it is so important to allow yourself to become comfortable with what you've learned here before moving on.

Chapter Four

Decision Counseling
for Spiritual Conflict

For many, spiritual conflict is a challenging topic of discussion. There are several reasons for this. First, counselors may not consider themselves to be adherents of a particular faith. They may not have grown up in a religious household nor been exposed to much religious teaching as children. Thus, they may feel poorly equipped to discuss religious concepts or relate to women who are feeling negative emotions as a result of conflict with their relationship to God. Second, for those who were raised in a religious context, they may not have fully worked through their own religion's opinions and beliefs about abortion. They may be afraid to find out what the leaders of their faith or place of worship believe. They may be apprehensive about feeling disappointed, rejected, or angry. Third, many may consider themselves spiritual, but not religious. They may not have had the opportunity to think about how spirituality can assist them in thinking through these issues.

Exercise 4.1

Take a moment to think about what *religion* means to you. What kinds of thoughts and feelings come to mind? What does *spirituality* mean to you? How is it different from religion? Write down your thoughts and feelings in your counseling journal.

How do we know when a patient is struggling with spiritual conflict? Consider the following four statements:

• I am afraid that God will not forgive me for having an abortion.
• I am committing a sin by having an abortion.

• I am worried that God will punish me in some way after the abortion.
• I am worried about what God thinks about me.

When you hear a woman express spiritual conflict, your initial reaction is quite possibly going to be fear, and in your fear you'll stop listening. You'll hear your patient say, "I think abortion is a sin, and I'm worried about what God is going to think about me." Your mind will promptly and dutifully freeze. You'll think to yourself, "Maybe it is a sin. I guess that's what she believes, so it doesn't seem like there's anything else I can say. This is pretty uncomfortable, so I'm going to find out whether she's sure about the abortion and move on to signing consent forms." The more that we accept that the patient has the answer to her dilemma, the less stuck we'll become when we hear spiritual conflict.

Exercise 4.2

Take out your counseling journal and write down some aspects of spiritual conflict that make you uncomfortable. This could be a list of things patients have said to you in the past or things you worry they *will* say. In addition to writing these down, describe *why* you find these particular statements challenging.

If you haven't given this issue a lot of deep thought, working with spiritual conflict can seem like a losing battle. When a patient says, "I'm afraid that God thinks abortion is a sin," your first thought may be, "Well, I guess God probably does," and find yourself lacking in anything else to say. Many helpful essays have been written about different religions' beliefs and teachings about abortion. A good place to start is to watch the videos by clergy from the Faith Aloud website. They are a testament to the breadth and depth of flexibility within religious belief. The next place to go is the website of the Religious Coalition for Reproductive Choice. Spend some time on this website and read the essays from the perspectives of different faiths; they will change the way you think about abortion and religion. In this chapter, I outline an approach and framework for working with patients who express spiritual conflict. My goal is to increase your confidence in these discussions and to broaden your thinking about the relationship between spirituality and abortion. The framework and approach are consistent with our work in chapter 3 on emotional conflict and contain the tools that you'll need to work within different situations.

Our fundamental principle, *the patient has the answer*, applies in the context of spiritual conflict and is the key to the counselor's success. Remember that the resolution of conflict, in particular spiritual conflict, can be found by the patient herself within her own beliefs and values. It is not your job to "solve" a theological dilemma. Presumably, you are not a rabbi, pastor, priest, or imam, so your task is not to offer absolution. You are there to help your patient unpack her own beliefs and look for the flexibility inherent within. Let's take a moment to review the three components of our *approach* in the context of counseling for spiritual conflict:

1. Listen.
2. Do not assume!
3. Self-reflect.

Be an active, engaged listener. This communicates interest and respect. Be curious about and genuinely concerned with the patient's well-being. If you are bored, afraid, distant, stiff, or judgmental when talking to a patient on the telephone or in person, she will instantly pick up on that and give it right back to you! You reap what you sow: the seeds that you plant in your approach to your patient determine what will grow between you. If you give respect and compassion, usually you will get it back. If you are interested in learning more about her, she will be more willing to share.

Don't assume that you and the patient share the same understanding of feelings and beliefs. This is especially true of language regarding spiritual and religious beliefs. Seek to understand how *she* understands the different religious concepts that she uses. The most important message that you need to take from this chapter is that you do not have to be an expert in the patient's religion. There are several important concepts that you and the patient can discuss together to explore *her* beliefs. The crux of the ability to converse fluently around spiritual conflict requires openness on the part of the counselor to become a student—in that moment—of the patient's religious or spiritual beliefs. You will learn from her, and she will learn from herself. We habitually forget our fundamental principle and our approach. We find ourselves in the paralysis of professional mode, where we feel the pressure to have all the answers. Who says that you can't be curious and explore your patient's words? Who says that you need to have the answer to her question and immediately solve her problem? Be interested in and fascinated by her dilemma. Wonder about what she's feeling. When we allow our minds to open, we free ourselves to ask these kinds of questions and listen carefully for the answers. Finally, self-reflect on what religion and spiritual conflict mean to you. Complete exercises 4.1 and 4.2 before reading further.

Let's take a moment to look a little deeper into the second part of our approach: not assuming. Being an interested, respectful listener is essential as you learn more about spiritual conflict and begin, possibly for the first time, to think about religious belief in a more philosophical way. Many counselors get stuck on the premise that if someone expresses a certain religious belief, they're probably unable or unwilling to question it. We trip up on the assumption that there is an inherent absence of flexibility regarding statements of belief and that there is no room for questioning, curiosity, or change. I think that sometimes we lend an unnecessarily stoic and distancing reverence to statements of religious belief instead of leading with the same inquisitiveness and openness that we cultivate in the face of emotional conflict. What we forget is that religious doctrine has experienced tremendous transformation throughout history and that a principle of many religious traditions is exploration, curiosity, and questioning (Maguire 2001). For example, human beings have elevated certain passages of the Hebrew Bible and the New Testament to differing levels of importance depending on the historical, social, and political context in which they live. Hermeneutics, the art and practice of interpretation, is an approach to understanding the meaning of texts and has been especially important for many scholars in their understanding of the Bible. Part of the practice of hermeneutics is the inclusion of the many contextual elements that contribute to a text's meaning. This means that when we set out to understand the meanings and intentions of a text, we take into account the life and perspective of the author, the social and historical context in which he or she wrote, and the political struggles of the time, alongside many other factors (Addison 1989). Keep in mind that even the Catholic Church has changed its practices and proscriptions over time. The church may state that it was God who made the need for these changes known, but one could venture that this supports the argument that even God's mind can change!

It is important to note that the Bible does not contain any passages that relate to abortion per se. The closest reference is Exodus 21:22, which tells a story of two men who are fighting. One of them accidentally hits a pregnant woman, causing her a miscarriage but no other injuries. The man who causes the miscarriage is ordered to pay the woman's husband a fine. That's the extent of it. Of course, those who consider abortion to be murder can cite chapter and verse regarding God's opinion on *murder*, but considering *abortion* to be murder is an *opinion* that each human being is free to hold. The Bible contains many "rules" for living, but we don't always follow all of them. Just as the messages within the Bible are complex, our interpretations of their meaning have endured many permutations. It's not hard to imagine that there could have been a story in the Bible about a woman putting pebbles in her uterus to cause a miscarriage and God's wrath coming down on her entire village. Even if this were the case, I think it's still equally as likely that we'd have legal abortion today.

The methods of seeking and thinking that allow the greatest freedom are those that create an approach of openness and compassion in place of judgment and constriction. Therefore, I approach religion from a liberal religious perspective, philosophy from a phenomenological perspective, and psychology from a humanistic perspective. I encourage the reader to further explore different texts that increase the capacity for contemplative thought and being present in the moment. The simplest (and sometimes most profound) expression of this capacity in the setting of abortion counseling is the ability to listen without interrupting, to sit in the space of silence with another person, and to acknowledge suffering. A lot of people wonder whether an abortion counselor is qualified to discuss spiritual matters. The short answer is yes. The reason for that is because abortion counselors are not offering spiritual advice or making religious pronouncements; they are conducting decision counseling. We lead with the fundamental principle: that the patient has, within her beliefs, the resolution to her conflict. As we move through different counseling scenarios, I will give examples of counseling on each of the three levels in our framework (see box 4.1).

Box 4.1.   Framework

Level 1: Validate and normalize.
Level 2: Seek understanding.
Level 3: Reframe.

LEVEL 1: VALIDATE AND NORMALIZE

Start by offering reassurance through validation and normalization. Validation is important so that the patient knows you're not afraid to "go there" with her. Here are some examples of validating statements you can use:

- I'm hearing that this has been really hard for you.
- I can imagine that the concerns you have about God have made it harder to be here.
- That sounds like a big burden to carry around.
- Based on what you've said, I can see how this has been difficult for you.
- It sounds like your situation has been challenging in terms of your spiritual beliefs.

Let's look at an example of an exchange between a counselor and a patient where the counselor uses validation:

> *Patient:* I've been so torn up about this. What if God hates me? I've prayed a lot about it, but it hasn't made me feel much better.
>
> *Counselor:* I can see that you're really worried about what God thinks. That must be pretty stressful for you.

This patient expressed some very important concerns that she has about God, and her usual strategies have not thus far provided much comfort. The counselor's response shows the patient that she is listening and has recognized the significance of the patient's struggle.

Difficult spiritual feelings can make a person feel alienated and alone. Let the patient know that you've talked to people about this before and that you want to talk with her too. That's part of normalizing.

> *Patient:* I'm worried about what God is thinking.
>
> *Counselor:* You know, a lot of women that I talk to have concerns about God. Can you say more about what you are worried about?

By asking the patient to say more, the counselor moved to level 2. The next section teaches how to seek understanding of spiritual conflict.

LEVEL 2: SEEK UNDERSTANDING

In this section, we'll examine four manifestations of spiritual conflict. It is critical to engage your active listening skills so that you and the patient can unpack and explore her beliefs. Your questions will help her to think about her beliefs in the context of making the decision to have an abortion.

Case Example 4.1
Will God Forgive Me?

> *Patient:* I'm afraid that God won't forgive me for having an abortion.
>
> *Counselor:* I can imagine that this has made it harder for you to come here.
>
> *Patient:* Yes, it's been on my mind for a long time.
>
> Counselor: Can you say more about what you've been thinking?
>
> *Patient:* I'm worried about what God is thinking and whether or not I'll be forgiven.

Counselor: Let's talk for a moment about your beliefs; I'd like to learn more about them. What does your religion say about forgiveness?

Patient: Well, I believe that God forgives. If you pray and ask for forgiveness, God will forgive you.

Notice how the patient's statement actually contains the answer to her dilemma. Remember the fundamental principle of our approach: no matter what the problem, *the patient has the answer*. Thankfully, we don't have to have the answer; she has it. If God forgives, why is she worried that God won't forgive her? Discrepant statements (God will forgive you, but not me) can speak to deeper, more uncomfortable feelings (I'm not worthy of God's forgiveness), or they may be habitual statements that come from things we've been taught but haven't reflected upon (see box 4.2). If there are feelings that are getting in the way of the patient's believing that God will forgive *her*, you'll want to uncover those.

Box 4.2. Will God Forgive Me?

Some women believe that God will forgive others, but not them. The question "Will God forgive me?" may have less to do with a doubt in God's *capacity* to forgive and more with a concern that the patient will be exempt from the possibility of forgiveness. Learn about her understanding of forgiveness and how forgiveness is sought. What is getting in the way of being forgiven?

Counselor: Have you asked God for forgiveness?

Patient: Yeah, I've tried to pray and ask for forgiveness.

Counselor: How did you feel about it?

Patient: Better, I guess [*Looks down and away*].

Counselor: I can tell that there is something that is still bothering you. Can you put your finger on what it is?

Patient: I'm worried about what God thinks about me.

Counselor: Can you say more about what worries you?

In her body language and words, the patient reveals that there is something holding her back from feeling forgiven. One could imagine that the she is concerned about whether she is worthy of forgiveness. She may feel doubt over her own goodness or worry that aspects of her situation put her out of reach of God's love. Patients who feel guilt and shame about their abortions are sometimes worried that God's forgiveness has a loophole and that they might fall into it. They will be the exception; they will be the person for whom God's grace is not merited. Thus, in a typical conversation, I seek to understand the patient's resistance to accepting the love and forgiveness that she believes in. Follow the flow of her feelings and the rationale that she is giving for her fears and concerns. Part of what you are doing is unpacking her beliefs and asking her to explore inconsistencies in her statements.

You might feel confused when you hear your patient describe her belief in forgiveness and at the same time express concern that she will not be forgiven. When something doesn't seem logical, use it as an opportunity and opening for gentle exploration. Our goal is not to criticize her thinking but to let her know that we are listening carefully and we have heard something that is important and interesting. Sometimes I even lead with the statement, "I just heard you say something that I think is very important, and I'd like to ask you more about it." Here are some examples of ways to frame your questions when you hear discrepant statements:

- If you believe that God forgives when you ask for forgiveness, and you have asked God for forgiveness, what is getting in the way of you believing that God has forgiven *you*, too?
- If you believe that God is a loving God, what is getting in the way of you believing that God loves *you*, too?
- If you believe that prayer is a way of talking to God, what is getting in the way of you believing that God hears *your* prayers?

Fortunately, most people of faith believe that God is loving and merciful, that God forgives, and that prayer is a legitimate way to communicate with God (see box 4.3). Unfortunately, some of these very same people have negative views of themselves because they are having abortions. Although it is rare, I have met women who staunchly believe that God would forgive a murderer or a rapist but not a woman who has an abortion. If that is the case, you'll need to explore the feelings that are keeping her stuck in the beliefs that she is bad, unforgivable, or alienated from God, and what makes abortion so unforgivable.

Case Example 4.2
Abortion and Sin

Counselor: I can tell that there's something that is still bothering you. Can you put your finger on what it is?

Box 4.3. What is Forgiveness?

The concept of forgiveness is prominent in many religions. Those raised in a religious context likely can explain their understanding of God's role in forgiveness. In the Jewish faith, Yom Kippur—the Day of Atonement—is the holiest day of the year and the time for repentance and forgiveness. Christians have the life, death, and resurrection of Jesus Christ as the embodiment of forgiveness and salvation. Muslims have multiple attributes of God, including merciful, compassionate, and ever forgiving. The patient's interpretation of these religious concepts is one of the most important tools that she has for spiritual resolution. Begin by exploring her feelings and the personal meaning of her beliefs. When someone expresses concern over the possibility of forgiveness, I am interested in learning about how she understands forgiveness in the context of her religious or spiritual beliefs.

Patient: I'm worried about what God thinks about me.

Counselor: Can you say more about that?

Patient: I'm worried that he won't forgive me.

Counselor: I've talked to a lot of other women about their concerns about forgiveness. What do you believe about forgiveness?

Patient: I was always taught that God forgives you when you ask for forgiveness, as long as you are sincere and try to do better next time.

Counselor: Do you still feel that is true?

Patient: Yes.

Counselor: Let's look at something important that you've brought up here. If you believe that God forgives when you ask for forgiveness, and you have asked for forgiveness, what is getting in the way of you believing that God has forgiven you, too?

Patient: Because I think that abortion is a sin.

Counselor: What is your understanding of sin?

In case example 4.2, the counselor seeks to understand the patient's feelings, and begins an exploration of the personal meaning of her beliefs. By asking her about her understanding of forgiveness and sin, the counselor is learning from the patient (see box 4.4).

Box 4.4.   Abortion and Sin

Don't assume that you and the patient share the same understanding
of complex terms such as *sin*. Learn about her understanding of sin,
forgiveness, and atonement. If forgiveness is possible, can she seek it?
If not, what is getting in the way?

Exercise 4.3

It can be helpful to examine your own understanding of sin, even if you
are not a religious or spiritual person. Take a moment to write down your
thoughts about the meaning of sin in your counseling journal, even if you
don't personally believe in this concept.

The point of doing this exercise is not so that you can come up with a
solution for the patient. That would be contrary to our approach. Instead, it
is valuable to think about the concepts, feelings, and ideas that our patients
are struggling with so that we can have genuine empathy for their situation.
Otherwise, our interest may seem hollow.

Next, let's look at how the counselor learns about the patient's definition of
sin, how she thinks God treats sin, and her beliefs about God's expectations
for how humans are supposed to deal with their own sinfulness. Sin is a
concept that needs to be explored for each individual; don't assume that you
know what it means for the patient.

> *Counselor:* I feel like I'm getting a better understanding of your beliefs. God
> forgives others, but he might not forgive you. I can see why you are having a
> hard time.
>
> *Patient:* [*Nods*]
>
> *Counselor:* Can you say more about why God might not forgive you?
>
> *Patient:* Because I think that abortion is a sin.
>
> *Counselor:* What is your understanding of sin?
>
> *Patient:* Well, I guess it's something we do that disappoints God, or something
> we do that is wrong and that we shouldn't do again.
>
> *Counselor:* Okay. And what does your religion suggest that a person should do
> after realizing that he or she has sinned?
>
> *Patient:* Probably ask God for forgiveness, try to learn from it, and try to do
> better next time.

Counselor: That's interesting, because that sounds like what you are trying to do yourself.

Patient: I guess so.

Counselor: Why would you be an exception?

Patient: I don't know. I guess I just feel so bad about getting an abortion. I feel like I'm being selfish and that if I cared I would take responsibility and have the baby.

The counselor is doing a good job of asking the patient to define her terms in order to understand where she is coming from. She gently points out a discrepant statement and discovers a host of negative feelings that the patient has about herself and her decision. Notice how at that point the discussion moved from *spiritual* conflict to *emotional* conflict—the patient feels that she is being selfish. Often, the origin or source of spiritual and moral conflict is negative feelings directed toward oneself. Getting at those feelings requires a desire to learn about the patient's beliefs and a willingness to accompany her through the examination of her beliefs.

Sometimes patients ask us about *our* opinion of God, sin, or forgiveness. It is important to resist reassuring her (or condemning her!) with an explanation of your own beliefs. While you might be tempted to make her feel better, it's a temporary fix. She needs to think through and come up with her own plan for resolution and discover that the answer can be found in her own beliefs:

Patient: What do *you* think God thinks about abortion? Do you think that he'll forgive me?

Counselor: You know, I can tell that you are really wondering about what God thinks, and that's okay. I'm glad we're talking openly about it. Other women have asked me the same question. I think that it is important for us to figure out what *you* believe and what *you* need to be at peace with your decision—no matter which one it is—so that you can move forward with your life and be happy and healthy.

Let the patient know that it is normal and okay for her to be curious about your beliefs. Tell her that others have wondered about and asked you the same thing. After you explore her beliefs a little further and find out the source of her spiritual conflict (I'm not worthy of God's love; I feel so guilty), suggest resources on religion and abortion. You can give her links to websites or books and provide handouts for post-abortion coping. Sometimes women benefit from talking to a leader in a religious community either before or after the abortion.

Case Example 4.3
Will God Punish Me?

When patients are worried about punishment from God, they may be unsure about whether abortion is morally wrong or whether it is a forgivable sin (see box 4.5). They may be struggling with a sense of their own "badness" resulting from a deep-seated shame. Seek to understand why the patient feels like she deserves punishment and whether she'll continue to punish herself in some way after the abortion is over.

Box 4.5.   Will God Punish Me?

When women wonder, "Will God punish me?" they can be revealing uncertainties about the morality of abortion or God's mercifulness. It may also reveal that they are harboring negative feelings about themselves. Learn about the patient's understanding of God. Learn about her beliefs about abortion and her feelings about herself. What is getting in the way of receiving God's mercy?

Patient: I'm worried that God will punish me in some way after the abortion.

Counselor: What are you worried will happen?

Patient: I'm worried that God will kill my children.

Counselor: Do you mean the children that you already have at home?

Patient: Yes.

Counselor: In your beliefs, what is God like?

Patient: I think that God forgives, but that he also punishes as well.

Counselor: How have you seen him punish?

Patient: By making people's lives hard and their children's lives hard.

Counselor: Why would God do that to you?

Patient: Because abortion is a sin and it's not forgivable.

Counselor: Hmm. I'm really struck by what you are saying. It sounds like you are in a really tough bind here.

Patient: [*Nods*]

Counselor: Let me ask you, given that there could be some serious repercussions to you having an abortion, what got in the way of you continuing the pregnancy?

It is always a good idea to explore continuing the pregnancy when a patient presents little flexibility in her beliefs, and this counselor is doing so in a way that takes the patient's beliefs seriously. She also frames the question about continuing the pregnancy in a way that is gentle and nonjudgmental. You don't have to do it at this exact point in the conversation, but it would be important to check in with her on this issue eventually. We explore this technique in greater detail in chapter 6 on ambivalence. Also, this is an opportunity to find out her reasons for having the abortion. This will prepare you for reframing. It is possible that she will tell you that there is no way that she can continue the pregnancy and that adoption is out of the question. If that is the case, then you can see whether she is open to another way of thinking about herself and the abortion, as we did in chapter 3. If you decide to explore continuing the pregnancy at this point in the conversation, you'll need to return to the exploration of her beliefs about how abortion is an unforgivable sin.

Here's another way to continue this conversation:

Patient: I think that God forgives, but that he also punishes as well.

Counselor: How have you seen him punish?

Patient: By making people's lives hard and their children's lives hard.

Counselor: Why would God do that to you?

Patient: Because abortion is a sin that's not forgivable.

Counselor: What does *sin* mean to you?

Patient: It's something that we do that is wrong in the eyes of God.

Counselor: In your beliefs, is there room for forgiveness of sins?

Patient: Yes, but not for abortion.

Counselor: Are there other sins that aren't forgivable?

Patient: Probably, but right now I can only think of abortion.

Counselor: Did you grow up with that belief?

Patient: Yes.

Counselor: Were you taught that in church?

Patient: Yes.

Counselor: Do you attend a church right now that holds that same belief?

Patient: Yes.

Counselor: I wonder whether there is anyone at your church who has ever had an abortion.

Patient: There was a girl who had an abortion. They kicked her out of the church.

Counselor: What did you think about that?

Patient: I thought it was awful, but she knew the rules.

Counselor: Are you anticipating that you'll be kicked out as well?

Patient: I'll get kicked out. My family will be very upset. But I'm an adult so I'll take responsibility for it.

Counselor: There's one thing that I'm feeling that I want to share with you. I feel like you're resigned to the fact that something very bad is going to happen but that there's nothing you can do about it.

Patient: That's exactly it.

Counselor: I want you to know that I understand that you are here to have an abortion, but I want to ask you, what got in the way of you continuing the pregnancy?

Patient: I'm in no position to have another baby. I am struggling to take care of my son on my own. The father of my son is also the father of this baby and he's out of work and he's started to become abusive. I can't keep being tied to him. I need to get myself on my feet and get myself and my son into a better situation.

Counselor: I can see what you're saying—continuing the pregnancy would be far worse.

Patient: That's pretty much it. Now you can see where I'm coming from.

Counselor: I want to return to something that you said earlier—that abortion was a sin that was not forgivable. What about sins that *are* forgivable? How are those different?

Patient: Hmm . . . that's a good question.

At this point, the patient feels that the counselor has truly comprehended her conundrum. They have established a good rapport, in part due to the counselor's authentic desire to be a student of the patient's beliefs. It was important that the counselor acknowledge the enormity of what the patient was facing—almost certain punishment from God, excommunication from her church, and no option to continue the pregnancy. It is going to be a challenge to try to introduce another way to frame the abortion, but we'll do that on level 3. Since we learned that the patient feels there is no way that she can continue the pregnancy and parent, we'll offer her a different way to see her abortion decision.

In this example, the counselor didn't bring up adoption. Talking about continuing the pregnancy (and subsequently parenting or placing the baby for adoption) with patients who have come to the clinic for an abortion requires a great deal of sensitivity and tact on the part of the counselor. For some patients, it is important for us to acknowledge that they are here to have an abortion and that we are talking with them because we want to optimize their post-abortion emotional health—not talk them out of having an abortion. When I broach the subject of continuing the pregnancy, I always start with the option of continuing the pregnancy and *parenting*. If I propose adoption, I do it last. It depends on the demeanor of the patient and how receptive she is to talking about parenting. In the case of ambivalence (when the patient feels torn between parenting and abortion), I almost always bring up adoption. When a patient reveals *conflict* with her decision yet desires an abortion, I don't always take up adoption as a separate topic. Part of self-reflection is being aware of when we, as abortion counselors, might sound like we are trying to talk our patients out of the abortion—even when that's not what we intend!

To move to level 3, there are a couple of paths that this conversation could take. First, the counselor needs to complete the exploration of unforgivable versus forgivable sins in order to introduce the possibility of flexibility in beliefs. This might mean making a connection between abortion and the realm of forgivable sins. That way, the patient might be open to seeing her decision in a slightly more positive way. On the other hand, the patient may be completely resigned to two things: (1) she has no choice but to have an abortion; (2) she will be punished for having an abortion. Just for the moment, let's take these two statements as fact: the patient is going to have an abortion; she has expectations of punishment from God. Given this, what can the counselor do for her? If nothing else, help the patient make a plan for coping with her anticipated punishment. Thus, it would behoove the counselor to learn more about how the patient anticipates being punished. Maybe it will be only a temporary, one-time punishment. In that case, she could plan to do penance by helping out in her community or taking in a needy child. Will this punishment continue into the afterlife? Is she worried that she will go to hell? If so, that is a much more serious burden for her. How will she cope with it? The expectation of punishment from God is a perfect example of when not to assume. The punishment that she expects may be something that she can live with; you won't know unless you ask.

Exercise 4.4

Let's look at a patient's statement that represents spiritual conflict and an example of a counselor's response. Then let's examine how closely the counselor's response follows the fundamental principle, "*The patient has the answer.*" Write your thoughts in your counseling journal.

Patient: I'm worried that God won't forgive me for having an abortion.

Counselor: Well, I think most people believe that God is kind and loving. I'm pretty sure that God will forgive you. He knows that you are struggling, and he can see what is in your heart.

This is a pretty good example of the *counselor* having the answer! This counselor may have good intentions, such as wanting to reassure the patient, but she lacks curiosity about the patient's personal beliefs about forgiveness. The counselor skipped ahead and tried to resolve the patient's dilemma by inserting her *own* beliefs. This counselor may also be uncomfortable talking about spiritual issues. The skills that you are developing through completing the exercises in this chapter will give you the courage to enter into discussions that may make *you* a little uncomfortable, but they will increase your capacity to witness the patient's experience. Remember that the patient may be a little afraid, too.

Exercise 4.5

Let's look at a patient's statement that represents spiritual conflict and an example of a counselor's response. Let's then examine how closely the counselor's response follows the fundamental principle, *"The patient has the answer."* Write your thoughts in your counseling journal.

Patient: I believe that abortion is a sin and it's not forgivable.

Counselor: I can imagine that this concern has made it harder for you to be here. This is a valid concern and I want to honor that for you. What have you thought about continuing the pregnancy?

This response sticks with the fundamental principle, but possibly to a fault. The counselor respectfully acknowledges that the patient's beliefs are very important, but by quickly moving to talking about continuing the pregnancy, it sounds as if she treats them as fact. What if there is some flexibility in the patient's beliefs about sin and forgiveness? These could be explored before ruling out continuing the pregnancy.

Case Example 4.4
Abortion and Sin

When a patient expresses a negative belief so strongly and firmly, such as in exercise 4.5, it can be difficult to conceive of how there could be flexibility therein. Why did she come here for an abortion if she believes that it is an unforgivable sin? This is an understandable response if you take the patient's statements at face value. But what if there are exceptions to the rule? What if her religion contains the means of forgiveness or atonement? In the following example, the counselor takes a different path before exploring continuing the pregnancy. Let's see what happens when we inquire further into the patient's beliefs:

Patient: I believe that abortion is a sin and it's not forgivable.

Counselor: What is your understanding of sin?

Patient: I think that it is something that we do that is wrong in the eyes of God.

Counselor: Are some sins forgivable?

Patient: Sure.

Counselor: Which ones are those?

Patient: Those that don't involve killing or don't involve forsaking God.

Counselor: In your beliefs, how does a person obtain God's forgiveness?

Patient: They pray. They ask God for forgiveness.

Counselor: What do you think God does when someone prays for forgiveness for an unforgivable sin?

Patient: I'm not sure. . . .

Counselor: [*Silence*] That's something interesting to consider.

Patient: [*Contemplating*]

Counselor: There's another good point you made that I wanted to ask you about. Are there times when someone kills but God forgives them?

Patient: Yes, I suppose so.

Counselor: Can you think of an example?

Patient: I guess when someone kills someone by accident or to protect themselves.

Counselor: That makes sense. What about people who have killed other people on purpose and go to prison? We sometimes hear stories about how they ask for God's forgiveness and then are saved. Some of them talk about having a religious conversion while in prison. What do you think about that?

Patient: I believe that God forgives them.

Counselor: That seems like an example of where killing or murder could be forgiven. What do you think?

Patient: I guess I never thought of it that way, but it's true.

Counselor: I think your beliefs are really important. That's why I'm asking you about them. I sometimes find that when I talk with women about their beliefs, they find out that it might be possible for them to be forgiven, too.

Patient: [*Contemplating*]

Counselor: What could you do now or after the abortion to ask God for forgiveness?

This example demonstrates that avenues of flexibility in the patient's beliefs about God, forgiveness, and sin often abound. The counselor's interest in learning about the patient's religious beliefs is the engine that drives the conversation. This is just one example of the path of a conversation. No matter which path you take, never assume that you and the patient share the same understanding of religious concepts. Allow yourself to be pulled by respectful curiosity and a motivation to discover possibilities within her point of view that she hasn't connected to her own situation. Moving to level 3, we'll make the transition to reframing her decision as a positive one and her view of herself as a moral person. We'll use the same skills that we learned in chapter 3.

LEVEL 3: REFRAME

It is often very powerful for the patient when you reframe the abortion as a decision made out of care, love, compassion, or mercy as opposed to one made out of selfishness, sinfulness, or thoughtlessness. Reframing statements are part of the concept of purposeful normalization: abortion is not a sin that denies women access to God but is instead a loving, caring, compassionate decision. It is a moral decision. In the words of Darcy Baxter, MDiv, it can even *connect* women to their god.

- I can see that you are making this decision because you believe in the importance of being able to care for your children and you want to be the best parent that you can be.
- You have been telling me how you have many people that you take care of and that there are people in this world who need you. Part of your family values is being there for them, caring for them, and giving them everything that you want to give them. For you, having this abortion is part of making sure that you can continue to care for others in the way that is essential to their survival.
- I'm hearing that it is important to you that your baby not suffer anymore. That is a loving, merciful act.

Reframing must be preceded by seeking to understand the patient's feelings and beliefs. It is premature to make these statements directly following the patient's disclosure of her concern about a spiritual matter. Spend some time exploring and learning about the patient's experience and her spiritual concerns. Look for flexibility within the patient's beliefs. Ask her to explore discrepant statements. Why is *she* excluded from God's love or forgiveness? Why doesn't God understand *her* situation? These reasons sometimes point to feelings about herself. Learning about these feelings and about the circumstances in her life that lead to the decision to have an abortion set the stage for reframing.

Discussion about beliefs can reveal flexibility. This can include examples of exceptions to a more rigid belief system. Exceptions are examples of times when the patient can see abortion as morally sound or acceptable in her own eyes or the eyes of God. Sometimes patients have a negative feeling about themselves that initially excludes them from feeling forgiven or accepted by God. Explore that emotional conflict. Then see whether the patient can see herself as included in her own beliefs, even if it's only as an exceptional circumstance. As you set the stage for reframing, revisit the patient's reasons for the abortion. Make a connection between the patient's life circumstances and the circumstances in which she and God feel abortion is acceptable. Her life circumstances are what help her to reframe her view of herself and her decision in a more positive way. This is a similar technique to that which we used in chapter 3 when we used the circumstances of the patient's life as the ingredients to reframe the abortion decision. In spiritual conflict, you'll use her life circumstances plus flexibility in her beliefs as these ingredients. Your goal is to help her see herself as being *included* within her beliefs so she can see herself as okay and abortion as acceptable (see figure 4.1).

This discussion brings up the difficult issue of patients who come to see their abortion as acceptable but continue to condemn the abortions of other women. This is not the goal of seeking flexibility in beliefs, nor is it the ideal outcome of thinking about one's own circumstances as an exception. Ideally, conversations that discover flexibility within a patient's religious belief come to include *all* women who have abortions. When patients are

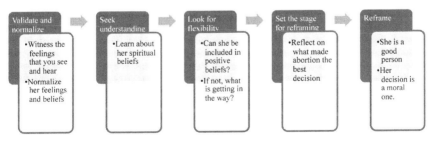

Figure 4.1. Decision Counseling for Spiritual Conflict

judgmental toward others because they don't seem contrite enough, I gently remind them that it is important to recognize that each woman has her own way of coping with her decision and how a person's outward behavior does not always represent her deepest feelings. I also remind them that they may in fact share life circumstances with some of the women in the waiting room. It is important for all of us to resist passing judgment until we have walked in another person's shoes.

Case Example 4.5
Abortion and Sin

In our earlier example about abortion and sin, the counselor spent some time at level 2 trying to understand the patient's definition of sin. In this segment, the counselor will introduce a reframe to offer a different way for the patient to think about herself and her decision.

Counselor: What does your religion suggest that a person should do after realizing that he or she has sinned?

Patient: Probably ask God for forgiveness, try to learn from it, and try to do better next time.

Counselor: That's interesting, because that sounds like what you are trying to do yourself.

Patient: I guess so.

Counselor: Why would you be an exception?

Patient: I don't know. I guess I just feel so bad about getting an abortion. I feel like I'm being selfish and that if I cared I would take responsibility and have the baby.

Counselor: Where do you think that's coming from, that feeling of selfishness?

Patient: I don't know, you know, a lot of people say that you shouldn't be able to "get out of being pregnant" by having an abortion. They say you should take responsibility and have the baby.

Counselor: I've heard women say that, too. What do you think that reveals about their feelings about pregnancy and having children?

Patient: I guess it's not very positive!

Counselor: It's interesting, isn't it? I want to go back to another thing you said. Some people tell me that they feel selfish about having an abortion. But other people tell me that having the baby would be selfish. It seems like what is "selfish"—and what is "taking responsibility"—is really a matter of opinion. You've told me a lot about your situation. You have three kids at home who need you to be able to care for them. You have a nine-month-old baby who needs your full attention. You are having an abortion because you need to be able to take care of the kids you already have. That sounds like a decision made out of love and care for others.

Patient: Yeah, I hear you.

Counselor: What do you think God thinks about your situation?

Patient: That there is no way that I can take care of another baby right now and also keep my family together.

Counselor: What do you think God thinks about *you*?

Patient: I think he understands my situation. I think he sees that I am struggling.

Counselor: What are some ways that you see yourself as a caring person?

Patient: Well, I'm caring for my three kids. I'm also caring on and off for my mother. She has a lot of health problems.

Counselor: That sounds like you are doing a lot of caring for others and have a lot of responsibilities.

Patient: I see what you are saying. Thanks for putting it that way.

Counselor: Part of feeling resolved spiritually is coming up with a plan for after the abortion. You mentioned earlier that part of your beliefs about forgiveness is learning from your mistakes and trying to do better next time. What could be part of that plan for you?

Patient: I could be more responsible the next time I have sex and make sure that I use birth control. I could make sure that he uses a condom.

Counselor: While I think that what you're saying is a good personal policy, I also want you to keep in mind that it takes two to tango—your partner has to take responsibility as well. Maybe part of doing better is also saying to yourself that you are a person of value, and that your partner needs to be concerned with your emotional and physical health and participate in birth control with you. If he cares about himself and about you he'll want to protect the both of you. What do you think about that?

Patient: I think that if I could do that, it would be a good change in my life.

In this example, the patient was very open to the way that the counselor reframed the concepts of *selfishness* and responsibility into *care* and responsibility. Readers who are interested in continuing to reflect on the moral dimension of decision making can turn to Carol Gilligan's *In a Different Voice* (1982). This text was a groundbreaking exploration of moral development in women and girls and the moral dimensions of decision making. Gilligan's conclusions were drawn in part from a sample of women making pregnancy decisions.

Whenever patients criticize their use (or nonuse) of birth control, I want to mitigate their self-blame by normalizing birth control failures and reminding them that successful contraception involves men *and* women. I also want to screen for intimate partner violence and birth control sabotage, such as a partner taking her pills away or poking holes in condoms. If this is the case, I assess her safety, create a plan of action with her, and talk to her about more "hidden" birth control methods such as injections, implants, or intrauterine contraception.

Case Example 4.6
Will God Punish Me?

Sometimes, patients have more ominous ideas about God's intentions. They may worry that God will punish them afterward. They may believe that they will never make it to heaven. They may even feel that God has specific malicious intentions, such as killing their children or making them infertile. These beliefs can cause much suffering and need to be explored further.

When you and your patient feel stuck, you can ask her how she feels about people who take a different perspective on the principles and practices within her religion. You may be able to remind her that there are people within her religion who are pro-choice. You'll gain more confidence around this issue after you become more familiar with the organizations Faith Aloud and the Religious Coalition for Reproductive Choice. You can also ask whether the patient has ever known anyone who was an independent thinker regarding religious practice or belief and how she felt about this person. These lines of questioning explore the possibility of flexibility in her beliefs. For example, many Catholics are fully aware of the pope's views on contraception but have decided to make their own decisions in this regard. Yet they still consider themselves to be Catholic. In the following dialogue, recall that when the counselor talked with this patient at level 2, she concentrated on getting a full understanding of her beliefs about God and punishment.

> *Counselor:* There's one thing that I'm feeling that I want to share with you. I feel like you're so resigned about this. Like something very bad is going to happen, but that there's nothing that you can do about it. You've said that continuing the pregnancy would be far worse, so you feel that you have no choice.
>
> *Patient:* That's pretty much it. Now you can see where I'm coming from.
>
> *Counselor:* Have you ever known other people of faith who thought differently about sin, forgiveness, and God's mercy?
>
> *Patient:* I guess so.

Counselor: Can you think of any examples?

Patient: Yeah. My aunt doesn't go to our church. She says she has her own beliefs and is close to God in her own way.

Counselor: What do you think about that?

Patient: I think that she's probably a lot happier now than she was when she went to our church.

Counselor: Do you see her way of being spiritual as a possibility for you?

Patient: Maybe a little bit.

Counselor: What part of your aunt's way do you think you could try out?

Patient: Maybe believing that God is more open-minded than what they teach at our church.

Counselor: If you believed that, how would it affect your feelings about your current situation?

Patient: I guess I'd feel less judgment from God.

Counselor: According to your aunt, what would God say about your situation?

Patient: He would look at my situation and know that I have no choice. I have kids right now that I'm struggling to take care of. I lost my job, and I'm trying hard to survive on my own.

Counselor: What might he say about forgiveness?

Patient: I guess he would say that I can be forgiven, especially if I try to make up for it by helping someone else in need, or helping a child.

Counselor: That sounds like a really good plan. What do you think about this new way of thinking about God?

Patient: I like it, but I won't be able to completely change my way of thinking just like that.

Counselor: What might help you get a start on this new way of thinking?

Patient: I guess talking to my aunt.

Counselor: That sounds like a good idea. Does she know that you are here today?

Patient: No, but I think that I could tell her. She was furious when they kicked that girl out of our church.

Counselor: It sounds like she might be a safe person to talk to. I'd also like to give you the number of a talk line where you can speak with clergy who have a different way of thinking about God and abortion.

This conversation revealed that the patient had more flexibility than previously thought. She also formed a post-abortion coping plan. When patients are in crisis, I will offer them privacy so that they can pray, meditate, or make a phone call to a spiritual leader if that would help. I also offer the opportunity to watch a video of Reverend Rebecca Turner or another clergy member from Faith Aloud. Because this patient initially anticipated an extremely negative reaction from God, it is important to check back in with her to see whether that has changed.

> *Counselor:* We've been talking for some time now, but one of the first things you said was that you were worried that God would punish you by killing your children. How are you feeling now about that possibility?
>
> *Patient:* I guess I don't feel like he will actually do that. It's just that I've always been told about the consequences of God's anger.
>
> *Counselor:* I understand that's been a strong message in your life. There are a lot of people of faith who believe in the strength of God's love and mercy. What do you think about that?
>
> *Patient:* I believe in that, too.

After staying with the feelings and unpacking the concepts, the counselor explores alternative ways of thinking from within the patient's life context. If the counselor hadn't spent time listening, the patient might not have felt compelled to listen back. That is why you sometimes need to stay at level 2 for a while.

Case Example 4.7
What Does God Think about Me?

Many patients have concerns about what God is thinking about them (see box 4.6).

Box 4.6.   What Does God Think about Me?

When a patient is worried about what God thinks about her, she may also be revealing her concerns about the judgment of others. Learn about her understanding of God and her relationship with God. Learn about her beliefs about abortion and her feelings about herself. What is getting in the way of God understanding her situation?

Patient: I'm worried about what God thinks about me.

Counselor: What do you think that God thinks?

Patient: Well, I think that he forgives me, but that he is disappointed in me.

Counselor: Can you say more about that?

Patient: Because I was irresponsible for getting pregnant and I didn't realize that I was pregnant for such a long time. I didn't want to have an abortion this late.

Counselor: What about having an abortion this late is hard for you?

Patient: I know how developed it is and that it looks like a baby. It makes me feel like I am killing a baby. How can I do this if I love children?

Counselor: What you are saying is very profound and very personal. There are a lot of women I talk to who struggle with this same issue. They feel like they know that abortion is the best decision, but actually *having* the abortion is such a hard thing to do.

Patient: That's exactly how I feel.

Counselor: Knowing that abortion is the decision that you need to make doesn't always mean that it is going to be an easy one. It's hard for a lot of people. What made abortion the decision that you needed to make?

Patient: My son is two, and he lives with his father. I love him so much; he's the reason that I'm trying so hard to get my life to a better place where I feel like I have a stable income and a stable place to live. My father left when I was very young. My sister and I moved back and forth between my mom and my dad, but neither of them had very much money to take care of us. It was hectic; I hated it.

Counselor: When I look at your situation, I see someone who is trying to make changes in order to help her child. You want your son's life to be better than your life was when you were his age. I've learned that women consider abortion *because* they love children and they care about what children need in order to be raised in a safe and loving environment. If you think about it that way, it is only *because* you love children that you would consider having an abortion. I hear you saying that you are trying to reduce and prevent the suffering of many people, including yourself, so that you can be a better mother.

Patient: I like the way that you think about it.

Counselor: You can think about it this way, too. I know that not everybody does, but lots of people do. You have the power to think about it in a positive way. Forgiving yourself and having compassion for yourself and your situation are the first steps toward being able to make a new start.

There are many healing statements that you can use to reframe the tremendous disappointment and feelings of failure that women have when they struggle with a pregnancy decision. First, draw their attention to the fact that "it takes two to tango." Responsibility for contraception is not solely the woman's; there was a man involved, and he could have insisted on using a condom. When relevant, help patients acknowledge that they were, in fact, using contraception, even if imperfectly. Second, use the patient's contraceptive history to reiterate some of the barriers that she has faced with contraception. Maybe she had side effects; maybe she had no money for a refill; maybe she asked for an intrauterine method but it wasn't covered by her insurance. There are countless examples of health system failures and other barriers that block access to contraceptives. At any rate, discourage continued self-punishment over contraceptive failure or contraceptive nonuse. Contraceptive methods aren't perfect, some are difficult to use, some aren't covered by insurance (some women don't even have insurance), and some cause side effects. On top of that, some women have partners who are abusive and sabotage their contraception in a deliberate effort to get them pregnant. Third, no one is perfect. We all make mistakes. That is part of being human. The best remedy is to make a plan of action so that things can be different next time. Self-blame and self-hatred aren't known for their effectiveness as agents of behavior change. Here's another way to reframe self-blame:

> *Counselor:* It's easy to blame ourselves when we get pregnant and we didn't want to, but you are human and we all make mistakes. Your body wasn't giving you signs that you were pregnant and you kept getting your period throughout. You counted on your body to let you know, and it didn't work out that way for you.

There are many resources that we can offer patients to develop a plan for spiritual resolution and think about their beliefs in a new way:

- Offer the opportunity to watch the videos with Reverend Rebecca Turner and clergy of different faiths on spirituality, religion, and abortion from Faith Aloud at http://www.faithaloud.org/. These videos are indispensable resources for helping patients toward spiritual resolution.
- Recommend the 1997 book *Peace after Abortion* by Ava Torre-Bueno at the website http://www.peaceafterabortion.com/. Torre-Bueno's book is a fantastic resource for coping with guilt, grief, and spiritual injury and for finding forgiveness and resolution.
- Give the patient a copy of "A Guide to Emotional and Spiritual Resolution after an Abortion" by Margaret R. Johnston and Terry Sallas Merritt, available from the Abortion Care Network website at http://www.abortion

carenetwork.org/. It is homework for ambivalent patients struggling with spiritual issues and a great resource for post-abortion coping plans.

- Give her a copy of "Spiritual Comfort: Before and after an Abortion" by Anne Baker and Reverend Annie Clark, available from the Hope Clinic website at http://hopeclinic.com/.
- Offer readings on the way that different religions, denominations, and churches view abortion from the Religious Coalition for Reproductive Choice website at http://rcrc.org/.
- Discuss the option of rescheduling her appointment after talking to a spiritual leader.
- Provide information on local congregations that are pro-choice.

FINAL THOUGHTS

The key to successfully talking about spiritual conflict is to release yourself from the obligation of having to know the answer to the patient's dilemma. Your task is to become a student of the patient's beliefs and to learn from her. If you have no background in religious or spiritual matters, don't panic. There are lots of resources for you to consult. Complete the exercises in this chapter in order to self-reflect on your own beliefs. That way, you'll become more aware of where you might get stuck.

No matter what your religious or spiritual background, prepare yourself to become open to and interested in what the patient is saying. Most of the time, a patient's beliefs provide the key to her spiritual resolution; you are simply guiding her through a reflection on her beliefs and asking her to honestly examine what is getting in the way of feeling like a good person who can be forgiven and who can remain close to God. If the patient feels that there is no flexibility in her beliefs yet is sure that abortion is the best decision for her, help her make a plan for coping after the abortion that includes readings, websites, talking to pro-choice leaders in the faith community, and counseling referrals.

It is my hope that you'll come to find discussions of spiritual conflict rewarding for both your patients and yourself. Talking with people about their spiritual beliefs, listening to and witnessing their fears and concerns, and working together to discover new ways of thinking about abortion to remove stigma and shame is revolutionary. You are part of an important movement that is trying to change the way women think about abortion and themselves. This is a gift for humankind.

Chapter Five

Decision Counseling
for Moral Conflict

Counseling patients with moral conflict about their abortion decision can be frightening, confusing, and overwhelming: the same patient who is resolute that she must have an abortion is equally adamant that abortion is murder or should be illegal. Some patients' ambivalence originates in moral conflict, but other patients with moral conflict are certain that they want an abortion. In addition, some women express their moral conflict with hostility, anger, and defensiveness. They may be outwardly and unabashedly rude toward clinic staff. They may attempt to distinguish themselves from other patients because they are not expressing sufficient sadness or regret for their decisions. These patients may seem completely unapproachable. However, many patients with moral conflict are open to an exploration of their feelings and their decision.

How do we know when a patient is struggling with moral conflict? Consider the following four statements:

• I really don't believe in abortion, but I have to do it.
• I believe that abortion is murder.
• I think that abortion should be illegal.
• I'm killing my baby.

When we hear such statements we find ourselves confused as to how to respond. Why would someone want to have an abortion if she really thought it was murder? How dare a patient ask us to provide her with an abortion while she continues to think of us as murderers? If abortion were illegal, then she wouldn't be able to have one! The confusion, anger, and fear that counselors feel when patients make these statements are normal. When moral conflict is expressed with hostility and defensiveness, the real challenge for the counselor is to support the patient without becoming offended or intimidated. It is important to keep in mind that outward expressions of anger and hostility are often a mask to conceal vulnerability or fear that is too overwhelming. The patient's anger is a defense against negative, self-directed emotions that arise from her conflict. Remember that for some people, it is easier to feel and express anger than fear, despair, shame, embarrassment, or humiliation. By validating and empathizing with the patient's situation, the skilled counselor can help her feel safe enough to express these more difficult feelings.

Other patients who reveal moral conflict are able to achieve resolution within the counseling session. Anger and hostility are often put forward as a defense against feeling difficult emotions such as sadness, guilt, loss, and disappointment. When a person feels that *all* of her emotions have been validated—the anger as well as the sadness—she may become open to discovering flexibility within her beliefs. Openness to a different way of thinking about herself and her abortion is part of a successful reframe. In this chapter we explore different techniques for working with moral conflict that follow our approach and framework.

Moral conflict raises important questions about patient autonomy to make medical decisions, providers' rights and responsibilities, informed consent, and consequences of less-than-optimal post-abortion emotional health. Providers may ask themselves, if a woman expresses extreme, inflexible moral conflict, is informed consent possible? What is my role (the clinic's role), if any, in preventing women from having abortions in these situations? How well can a woman possibly cope after her abortion when she feels that she has committed murder? How do her beliefs affect my view of myself as a health care provider, and am I comfortable with that? All of these questions are valid and important to explore for yourself and with your coworkers. Each clinic must decide its own policy regarding whether and how it will screen for, assess, and treat moral conflict. Each clinic must also decide the degree of resolution of moral conflict that is necessary before a provider will allow a patient to consent to an abortion. There are many opinions about and many practices for dealing with these cases. I have found that many different opinions and approaches have merit and that this is a decision that clinics must make based on their experience and values.

Exercise 5.1

Reflect on your opinions regarding moral conflict and its effect on you, patients, and the clinic. Take out your counseling journal and write down your answers to the following questions. It will be rewarding to return to your answers after you have completed the work in this chapter to see whether your feelings and thoughts have changed.

1. Without self-censoring, describe your approach for working with women who express moral conflict. Are you more likely to engage in or avoid a discussion about moral conflict with a patient?
2. How do you feel when a woman says, "I'm killing my baby?"
3. Do you think informed consent is possible when a woman says, "I believe that abortion is the same thing as murdering a newborn baby?" Why or why not?
4. If you were (or are) a clinician performing abortions, would you provide an abortion for a woman who told you that abortion . . . "is murder?" "Is immoral?" "Should be illegal?" Why or why not?
5. Is refusing to provide an abortion in any of the situations in (4) a barrier to accessing care? Why or why not?

In this chapter, I present case examples where patients' beliefs become more flexible as a result of discussion, as well as examples where patients remain hostile and defensive for quite some time. We can all think of examples of outspoken, aggressive patients who just want to "get it done" but also don't "believe in abortion" because abortion is murder, abortion should be illegal, or their abortions are somehow different from everyone else's. Often these patients are very disruptive in the clinic, leaving staff feeling angry, resentful, or afraid. Sometimes women express extreme negative beliefs because they are ashamed about having an abortion and want to separate themselves from others and even from their own actions or circumstances. They may perceive others as being morally inferior because they are not expressing enough guilt or regret for their decisions. Seeing other women talking or laughing with one another in the waiting room can seem heretical. How do we understand such behavior?

One of the most well-known theories in social psychology is the phenomenon of cognitive dissonance (Festinger, 1957). Cognitive dissonance is the experiential state that arises when there is conflict or disagreement between one's beliefs and one's behaviors. Because the state of experiencing this dissonance (think discord or a clashing of nonharmonious sounds) generally is unpleasant, people will go to lengths to avoid consciously experiencing it. A person has three choices. She can become more flexible and change her beliefs to be more aligned with her behaviors, become more flexible and change her behaviors so that they are more in sync with her beliefs, or strive to rationalize or justify her beliefs and her behaviors. In our case of moral conflict, it is in the latter situation—simultaneously maintaining her decision to have the abortion and her negative attitude toward abortion—that we can find ourselves unsure as to how to counsel her. On the other hand, many patients are interested in discussing their moral conflict and can do so without becoming angry or defensive. In counseling they may change their views about abortion to include the acceptability of abortion within their life circumstances. It is even more rewarding when patients come to express less judgmental views about abortion or women who have abortions. Becoming more flexible in one's beliefs or one's behavior helps to resolve cognitive dissonance.

Let's take a moment to review the three components of our *approach* in the context of counseling for moral conflict:

1. Listen.
2. Do not assume!
3. Self-reflect.

Be an active, engaged listener. This communicates interest and respect. Be curious about and genuinely concerned with the patient's well-being. If you are bored, distant, stiff, or judgmental when talking to a patient on the telephone or in person, she will instantly pick up on that and give it right back to you! You reap what you sow; the seeds that you plant in your approach to your patient determine what will grow between you. If you give respect and compassion, usually you will get it back. If you are interested in learning more about her, she will be more willing to share. Don't assume that you and the patient share the same understanding of feelings and beliefs. When a patient uses inflammatory words such as *murder* or *killing*, ask her to describe the personal meaning of those words; don't assume that you and she are on the same page. Finally, self-reflect on what moral conflict means to you in exercise 5.1.

As we move through different counseling scenarios, I will give examples of counseling on each of the three levels in our framework (see box 5.1). In our framework, validation occurs at level 1. Throughout this chapter, we will explore the importance of validation at many points in the conversation in order to acknowledge emergent feelings. Anger will grow like wildfire unless it is witnessed and validated. As anger dissipates, the wall of defensiveness comes down. Behind the anger are the feelings that the patient is working hard *not* to feel—sadness, disappointment, shame. Hostile, angry, and defensive patients are protecting themselves from feelings that are too overwhelming. They are not really angry at us. They deserve our empathy and compassion. At level 2, seek understanding. When a patient expresses feelings, follow the guidelines for working with emotional conflict. Seek understanding of the personal meaning of her feelings and their origins. Similarly, what do the words *murder*, *killing*, and *immoral* mean to her? What is it like to have those beliefs? Where do her beliefs come from? Are there exceptions? Her answers to these questions, plus her reasons that abortion is the best decision for her

```
┌─────────────────────────────────────────────────────────────┐
│                    Box 5.1.   Framework                      │
│                                                              │
│   Level 1: Validate and normalize.                           │
│   Level 2: Seek understanding.                               │
│   Level 3: Reframe.                                          │
│                                                              │
└─────────────────────────────────────────────────────────────┘
```

at this time in her life, set the stage for reframing at level 3. Reframing offers the patient a view of herself as a good person and abortion as a moral decision. Return to level 1 to validate any difficult feelings that emerge. Support her with all of your might.

LEVEL 1: VALIDATE AND NORMALIZE

Working with moral conflict presents the greatest challenge to the skill of validating and normalizing. First of all, you may become anxious upon hearing the patient's anti-abortion views. Second, you know that expressing extremely negative views of abortion while at the same time demanding an abortion is *not* normal. However, you can communicate that other women have made similar statements about abortion and that your intention is to understand their personal meaning. Validate the patient's anger by empathizing with the difficulty of her situation. When you uncover the difficult feelings underneath the anger, recognize them. Acknowledge the patient's strength and courage for sharing them with you. Moral conflict requires significant effort in order to establish and maintain rapport. Use the first component of our approach—*listen*—as your guide. Respectful listening can persuade a patient to let go of anger and share difficult feelings.

Case Example 5.1

Counselor: What was it like for you to make the decision to have an abortion?

Patient: [Defensively] Well, I'm against abortion. I think that it's morally wrong and I think that it should be illegal.

Counselor: I appreciate your honesty. It must be really hard for you to be here.

Patient: [More relaxed] Yeah, it's hard, but I have to do it.

Counselor: I've talked to other women who expressed similar beliefs. I'd like to get a better understanding of what that means for you and your life situation.

When you say that you think abortion is morally wrong, can you say more about what you mean by that?

Validating this patient's anti-abortion views was captured in two sentences: "I appreciate your honesty. It must be really hard for you to be here." Normalizing was achieved by "I've talked to other women who expressed similar beliefs." Then the counselor moved toward gaining a deeper understanding of the patient's beliefs. Validating the patient's negative opinion about abortion helps to prevent defensiveness. It also shows that the counselor is not shocked or frightened by what the patient is saying. She truly wants to understand the patient's position. "It must be really hard for you to be here" also communicates that the counselor is aligned with the patient's desire to have an abortion.

Exercise 5.2

When talking with patients who are angry, hostile, or defensive, it will be important to use a neutral tone of voice and composed facial expression. If validating an angry patient does not result in a respectful exchange, you will have to speak firmly and match her energy to communicate that abusive language directed toward staff or other patients is unacceptable. In this exercise, pair up with a friend or coworker. Practice making these statements in a serious and self-confident way. You may need to say them several times in order to feel comfortable. Each time you practice, say them more firmly and unwaveringly.

- Thank you for sharing your feelings with me. I appreciate your honesty. I can imagine that it must be hard for you to be here.
- Given your beliefs, I can see how this has been a tough decision for you.
- I appreciate that you've been straightforward with me. I'll need you to bear with me for a moment because I need to ask you a couple of questions. This is part of our protocol at the clinic.
- I can see why you were upset in the waiting room. Keep in mind that different people cope with their experience in different ways.
- I appreciate you sharing your opinion, but please know that at this clinic we think about abortion in a different way.
- You're expressing some views that are not particularly complimentary about the work that we do here at this clinic. I'm going to commit to hearing out your views, but I'll expect that you'll treat me the way that you would expect me to treat you—with respect.

LEVEL 2: SEEK UNDERSTANDING

Exercise 5.3

It can be alarming the first time that you hear a patient use the word *killing* in reference to her abortion. It is important that we take time to explore our own thoughts around the meaning, purpose, and place of abortion in the life cycle. In this exercise, find a quiet place to think and write in your counseling journal.

1. Describe the *purpose* of abortion as if you had to explain it to someone visiting from another planet.
2. How would you define *killing*? How is it different from *murder*?
3. What are the contexts in which killing is acceptable in our society?
4. Are we more accepting when men kill than when women kill? Why or why not?

You may come to find that most patients use the word *killing* to acknowledge that abortion unambiguously terminates a pregnancy from growing, ends a potential life, or ends life. *Kill* may feel technically accurate to the patient. It may or may not be an indicator of moral or emotional conflict about abortion. You won't know unless you ask. The same is true about the word *murder*. Merriam-Webster Online defines murder as "the crime of unlawfully killing a person especially with malice aforethought." Furthermore, Merriam-Webster states that as a verb, murder "specifically implies stealth and motive and premeditation and therefore full moral responsibility." It would be unusual to meet someone who felt malice, negative intentions, or badness in her heart toward the fetus, therefore wanting to kill it. This is usually the point at which most people separate their definitions of what they are doing from murder. Most patients do not think they are committing a crime, nor do they possess "malice aforethought." That is an important nuance between murder and killing; technically speaking, to kill "merely states the fact of death caused by an agency in any manner." Abortion will stop the pregnancy from growing; it terminates the process of development of an embryo or fetus. That is the aim of abortion. For some, killing is the best way to describe this fact. The word *murder* is associated with more negative feelings than killing. Explore what it means for your patient. Is it the same as killing a newborn baby? Is it the same as killing an adult person? Does she expect to be prosecuted criminally after this abortion? If she actually believes it is murder, how does she expect to cope afterward while carrying this burden?

Look back at your answers to question 1 in exercise 5.3. What words did you use? What words did you avoid using? Why? Remember that most patients do not use inflammatory language, so you are investigating something that is meaningful in part because it is not typical. Behind your interest in or concern with the patient's word choice is the motivation to ensure that she is certain about her decision and can cope post-abortion. You can share this motivation with your patient. Your interest also reminds her that you are listening carefully to what she is saying. She may not be accustomed to this level of attention, and it can be affirming. I've found that some people use inflammatory words quite casually. I've had patients say to me in the most informal manner, "So do they kill the baby today with the seaweed?" It no longer shocks me, but I let patients know that I am paying attention.

> *Counselor:* I just want to check in with you. You used a word (phrase, expression) that means different things for different people. When you said that it feels like you are killing your baby, what do you mean by that?

Much of the time, women will explain that they just mean ending the pregnancy or stopping a life from growing. They do not think of themselves as having malice in their hearts or bad intentions. Exploring the patient's use of the words *killing* and *murder* becomes an important segue into an exploration of any emotional conflict that may reside underneath.

Case Example 5.2

> *Counselor:* I want to ask you about something that you said earlier. You used the word *murder* to describe how you feel about abortion. What does that word mean for you?
>
> *Patient:* For me, it's the same as if I killed one of my kids.
>
> *Counselor:* I can see the seriousness of this for you. Let me ask you another question: When people use the word *murder*, they sometimes are describing someone who is acting with malice or bad intentions. Does that sound like how you feel?

At this point, the patient may take a step back to explain that it's not that she feels any ill will toward the baby, only that she is struggling with the morality of her decision. As the counselor asks her to say more and seeks understanding of her feelings, the patient may reveal that she is struggling with guilt and sadness. If a patient can get in touch with her feelings, then she is more receptive to support and reassurance and a reframing of her decision.

Patient: [*Starts to cry*] I don't have bad feelings in my heart toward the baby, but I think that this *is* a baby. I'm killing her—I'm letting you guys kill her, but I have to!

Counselor: It's okay to cry. What feelings are coming up for you right now?

Patient: [*Crying*] I feel guilty.

Counselor: You are really brave to share your true feelings. Do you know where the guilt is coming from?

Patient: The baby is innocent. I am making a decision to kill her, and that makes me responsible.

Counselor: That sounds like a really heavy burden for you to carry around.

Patient: [*Sniffling*] It is.

Counselor: Maybe I can offer a way to see your decision differently.

Patient: [*Dries her eyes*] Okay.

Counselor: Tell me, what is going on in your life that made abortion the decision that you needed to make?

In case example 5.2, the patient's moral conflict gave way to reveal emotional conflict. The counselor sought to understand the patient's feelings and their origins. She validated the patient and supported her as she cried. The patient responded by indicating that she was open to a new way of thinking about her decision. To review, there are three components of seeking understanding of feelings or beliefs. Let's look at some additional ways to phrase those inquiries, specifically in the context of beliefs. First, seek understanding of the *personal meaning* of the patient's choice of words.

- I'm interested in getting a better understanding of what the word *immoral* means to you.
- If abortion were illegal, what would that mean to you?
- I'd like to better understand your beliefs. When you say that abortion is wrong, what does that mean to you?

Second, ask the patient what it is like for her to have her beliefs. This question gives the patient the opportunity to describe further what it is like for her to be anti-abortion and yet seek abortion care. Her answers may provide you with another opportunity to validate her struggle. This will help you to build rapport.

- What is that like for you, to wish that abortion were illegal?
- What is that like for you, to believe that abortion is immoral?

• What is that like for you, to feel that abortion is wrong but still need to have one?

Or just simply, "What is that like for you?" Third, seek an understanding of the *origin* of a patient's beliefs. This is similar to seeking an understanding of the origin of a feeling. Understanding the origin of a patient's beliefs about abortion provides another avenue from which to seek flexibility in her beliefs.

• Growing up, what did you think about abortion?
• How have you thought about abortion throughout your life?
• How did you come to your beliefs about abortion?

The personal meaning and origin of a patient's beliefs are platforms for reframing. Within them, the counselor can look for places of flexibility in the form of *exceptions*. Even women who are anti-abortion are usually able to pinpoint examples of when abortion is acceptable. Many times, those exceptions turn out to be quite similar to the patient's own situation. Your job is to make this connection and to see whether she can become open to including herself and her decision in the realm of the acceptable. It is important to keep in mind that there are times when patients are *not* open to discovering new ways of thinking about the abortion. Counselors often feel stuck when they find themselves in these situations. Some patients teach us that there really isn't anything we can do for them even though they appreciate the effort.

Case Example 5.3

Patient: I feel like I'm killing my baby.

Counselor: That must make it hard for you to be here.

Patient: Yeah, but it's what I have to do.

Counselor: What does that mean for you, to feel like you're killing your baby?

Patient: Well, it means that I am making a conscious decision to end a life. That I am taking responsibility for killing a baby that I don't want to have, that I don't want to be born.

Counselor: What is that like for you?

Patient: Well, I feel bad. I really wish I didn't have to do this, but it's what I have to do.

Counselor: How have you thought about abortion throughout your life?

Patient: Pretty much this same way. I never thought I would be in this situation. But I am, and I know what I need to do.

Counselor: I can tell that you are really clear about what you need to do. I want you to know that the motivation behind my questions is to see whether there's a way I can help you feel better about yourself or your decision.

Patient: I don't really think that there's a way for you to help me, although I appreciate that you want to try. This is just the way I think about it.

Counselor: Okay. Then let's come up with a plan for after the abortion in case you want to reach out to someone.

Patient: I don't think I'll really need it.

Counselor: You're right; you might not need it at all. If it's okay with you, I'm going to put a couple of cards in your to-go bag that have the numbers of free talk lines for after the abortion. Also keep in mind that you can always call here to talk to me or any other counselor.

Patient: That's fine.

Counselor: I get the impression that you are very sure about your decision. Also, you seem to know yourself well and know what you can handle. I don't mean to imply that you won't be fine afterward—I ask everyone these questions to see whether there is a way that I can help. If someone doesn't need my help, that's okay, too.

Patient: I understand. I know that you're just doing your job.

In the next section, we'll look at several different case examples. In each one, the counselor will begin by seeking understanding of the patient's beliefs or feelings. In case examples 5.4 and 5.5, the counselor will guide the patient through an examination of her feelings and beliefs, find flexibility, and offer a reframe. In case example 5.6, the counselor will look for flexibility in the patient's *decision*; in other words, she will explore the possibility of continuing the pregnancy. Finally, in examples 5.7–5.10, we will look at some challenging cases in which the patient has some significant hostility and defensiveness. Validation will help lessen anger and allow the counselor to move toward a reframe.

LEVEL 3: REFRAME

Figure 5.1 illustrates the flow of the conversation when counseling for moral conflict. This flow represents the path toward reframing the patient's view of herself and her decision. Each of the three levels of our framework is present. Because moral conflict involves beliefs that are anti-abortion to different degrees, the counselor needs to take time to explore those beliefs and look for flexibility. Find exceptions and see whether the patient is amenable to

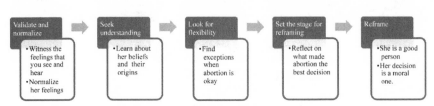

Figure 5.1.   Decision Counseling for Moral Conflict

seeing her own situation as an exception. To accomplish the reframe, reflect back her reasons for the abortion (why abortion is the best decision for her given the circumstances of her life). Use her life circumstances to reframe the abortion decision as loving, caring, merciful, or compassionate. Reframe the patient's sense of herself as a person who is trying to care for others or as a person who cares about the welfare and well-being of children. If reframing fails, make a plan for coping after the abortion.

Flexibility in Beliefs

Discovering flexibility in beliefs is the key to a more positive, inclusive view of abortion. First seek to understand the patient's beliefs about abortion and the origins of those beliefs. In any given situation, a person's beliefs—and the judgments that stem from them—will be either in conflict with or congruent with her behaviors. Remember what we learned about cognitive dissonance. When our planned behaviors are in conflict with our beliefs, we don't feel so good about ourselves. Most people leave room for *exceptions* to the more rigid *rules* they strive to live by. Our goal here is to see whether the patient's beliefs allow for exceptions and whether her situation fits into one of those exceptions. In other words, is she able to reconcile her own situation within a more flexible belief system?

Case Example 5.4

Counselor: So what was it like for you to make the decision to have an abortion?

Patient: It was hard, really hard.

Counselor: What made it hard?

Patient: I believe that abortion is wrong.

Counselor: Can you say more about your beliefs?

Patient: Well, I grew up being taught that abortion was wrong.

Counselor: Can you say more about what you mean when you say that abortion is wrong?

Patient: Just that it's immoral.

Counselor: What's that like for you?

Patient: It sure makes it hard to have an abortion.

Counselor: I bet it does. Can you say more about where your beliefs come from?

Patient: What do you mean?

Counselor: I guess I'm trying to understand whether your beliefs come from something that you believe God thinks, or whether it comes from something that people think, or both.

Patient: I think that God thinks it's immoral, so people should, too. My parents are against it, and our church always talked about it.

Counselor: Have you always thought this way about abortion?

Patient: Yes.

Counselor: I can see how that made this decision hard. Have you ever thought about examples of different situations where abortion is not wrong?

Patient: Maybe there are some. . . .

Counselor: What are some of those?

Patient: Well, when a woman is raped, or is being abused, or doesn't have enough money to raise a baby. . . .

Counselor: What about these situations makes abortion different for you?

Patient: Well, I guess it's because the woman is caught in a tough situation and she has no other way out.

Counselor: I wonder if some of the situations where you say that abortion is not wrong might be similar to your situation.

Patient: I guess some of them are.

Counselor: What are some of the things that are similar?

Patient: Well, I'm still in high school and I have no way to support myself or a baby.

Counselor: What else?

Patient: There's no way that I can take care of a baby right now.

Counselor: Have you ever thought about how having an abortion could be a moral decision?

Patient: What do you mean?

Counselor: It seems like you are deciding to have an abortion because it's not the right time to have a baby. You want to be able to give a baby the kind of care that it needs. Having an abortion lets you be able to plan for a baby later and provide it with everything that you think is right. It's a moral decision because you are thinking about what is fair and just for everyone involved. Do you think it's possible to see it that way?

Patient: [*Thinking*] Yeah. . . .

Counselor: What about God? Do you think it's possible that God sees it as a moral decision, too?

Patient: I suppose so.

Counselor: How so?

Patient: I believe that God knows what is in our hearts and what we are going through.

Counselor: That's a nice way of looking at it. It seems like you have discovered how abortion can be a decision that is made out of care and concern for others and for yourself. That is what I have learned from talking to girls here at the clinic. Do you think that you could see your own decision in that way?

Patient: You know, I actually could think about it that way. Thank you.

In this example, the counselor reframed the patient's view of herself and her abortion decision. She started by seeking understanding of the personal meaning of the patient's use of the word *immoral* and then asked her what it was like for her to believe that abortion was immoral. Not surprisingly, the patient said that it made it harder to have an abortion. The counselor then explored the origin of the patient's beliefs and discovered that they came from her family and her church. Next, she investigated whether there was any flexibility in the patient's beliefs. In other words, were there times when abortion did not seem immoral? She then added the ingredients of the patient's life situation. The patient's beliefs about abortion were actually more flexible than originally assumed, because she could envision how her own situation was similar to a situation where she believed abortion was acceptable. In the end, the patient was open to a reframing of abortion as a decision made out of the care and concern for others.

Flexibility in Feelings

Discovering flexibility in feelings is another avenue to reframing moral conflict. Sometimes, our exploration of patients' use of inflammatory words reveals that they're not using words like *murder* literally. Instead, these words reveal difficult emotions that are present for them in making the decision to have an abortion. In a way, these particular patients are more similar to patients who are experiencing emotional conflict.

Case Example 5.5

Counselor: When people use the word *murder*, they sometimes mean to say that someone is acting with malice and bad intentions. Is this how you feel?

Patient: [*Starts to cry*] I don't have bad feelings in my heart toward the baby, but I think that this *is* a baby. I'm killing her—I'm letting you guys kill her, but I have to!

Counselor: It's okay to cry. What feelings are coming out for you right now?

Patient: [*Crying*] I feel guilty.

Counselor: You are really brave to share your true feelings. Do you know where the guilt is coming from?

Patient: The baby is innocent. I am making a decision to kill her, and that makes me responsible.

Counselor: You are in a really tough situation. Maybe there's a way for me to help you see your decision differently.

Patient: [*Listening*]

Counselor: I'm hearing that you feel that way, but I wonder if there's another way to look at it. What if you thought about the abortion as a way of being compassionate toward this baby that you love but cannot have? You've made it clear that you've looked at your life and determined that you cannot take care of another child right now. You've finally found a good job and you need it in order to provide for your family. That's about caring for others. You are a good person trying to lessen the suffering of everyone, including the baby. When it's the right time for you to bring a child into this world, you'll know.

Patient: [*Sniffling*]

Counselor: Does that fit with how you think about yourself?

Patient: Yes.

Counselor: You're a good person and you're trying to do the best that you can.

Patient: Thank you.

Seeking Flexibility in the Decision

When someone expresses extreme, negative views about abortion but at the same time is demanding an abortion, I seek to understand her reasons *for* the abortion and *against* continuing the pregnancy. In other words, what brought her to the clinic? While I wouldn't frame the question as a "why?" question, my intent is the same. I want to understand what brought her to the clinic and how she envisions abortion as her best alternative despite her strong anti-abortion beliefs. While seeking flexibility in her decision, a patient may realize that continuing the pregnancy actually is an option for her. Or, she may remain adamant that continuing the pregnancy is impossible. If that's the case, I use her life situation to offer a reframe.

Case Example 5.6

Counselor: So what was it like for you to make the decision to have an abortion?

Patient: Well, I don't really believe in abortion, but I have to do it.

Counselor: What do you think about abortion?

Patient: Well, I think that it's taking an innocent life.

Counselor: That must have made it hard to come here today.

Patient: Yeah, it was hard.

Counselor: Where did your beliefs about abortion come from?

Patient: I've always been against abortion. Everyone in my family is. If you get pregnant, it's your responsibility. You don't just get to undo your mistakes and get rid of it.

Counselor: Sounds like you have pretty high standards for personal responsibility.

Patient: I do.

Counselor: Can you think of examples where you've thought that abortion was acceptable?

Patient: Not really.

Counselor: Hmm. Are there times when you've understood why a woman might have an abortion even if she were against it?

Patient: Maybe a woman who was raped. I could see why she would want to do it, but I would still think it was wrong.

Counselor: I see what you're saying about your beliefs. For you, it's pretty black and white. Abortion is wrong, no matter what the circumstances.

Patient: That's pretty much it.

Counselor: I can imagine that someone with your beliefs would think long and hard about continuing the pregnancy. What's made continuing the pregnancy impossible?

Patient: There's no way I can have a baby right now.

Counselor: How so?

Patient: I'm not ready. I don't have a job or any money. The father is completely irresponsible and he has pretty much disappeared.

Counselor: It sounds like it wouldn't be a good situation for you or for a baby.

Patient: No, it wouldn't.

Counselor: It seems like in some ways there's an aspect of having this abortion that's about taking responsibility for the situation.

Patient: What do you mean?

Counselor: I guess I'm looking at the concept of responsibility in a different way. Having a baby when it's *not* the right time or the right situation is not necessarily the best way to take responsibility. It just seems like you'd be punishing yourself for getting pregnant by having the baby; that also ends up punishing the baby.

Patient: I hadn't thought of it that way.

Counselor: It might be helpful for you going forward to think about it that way.

In the segment above, the counselor validates the difficulty of the patient's decision to come to the clinic despite her beliefs and then seeks to understand the origin of her beliefs. Next she explores the flexibility of the patient's beliefs and looks for circumstances where she might think abortion is acceptable. At first glance, this patient seems to have fairly rigid beliefs. But by taking another look at her life situation, the counselor put forward a different way to see her decision. When seeking flexibility in a patient's *decision*, it is imperative that your tone of voice be neutral and free of judgment. Practice ways to finesse your phrasing and timing of questions so that the patient doesn't think that you're trying to interrogate her or to make her justify why she isn't having a baby. Through your tone of voice and phrasing you are communicating that you: (1) understand that she is here for an abortion, (2) take her beliefs seriously, and (3) are motivated to help her plan for coping.

Counselor: Thanks for sharing all these feelings with me. I appreciate your honesty. Can I just ask you, what got in the way of your continuing the pregnancy?

This style of phrasing is purposeful. It is a check-in, not a request for justification. If she responds that she doesn't want to talk about it, then you don't need to push. You can also be transparent that her ability to access services is not in jeopardy.

Counselor: You are still going to be able to have the abortion today. I want to check in on a few things that you said so that we can come up with a plan for taking care of yourself after the abortion.

This statement can go a long way toward preventing the patient from becoming more defensive or closed down because she is worried that the clinic might deny her an abortion. Many patients who are angry, hostile, and defensive also are very certain about their decision to have an abortion. Their certainty contributes to their hostility. They may feel that they "have no choice" but to have an abortion. They may be defending against shame, embarrassment, humiliation, and fear. They sometimes also state that they wish abortion were illegal. Paradoxically, they wish it were illegal *right now*, and then they wouldn't be able to get one. They are overwhelmed with the thought of taking responsibility for and ownership of the decision. They resent their right to choose because it is too overwhelming to assume responsibility for something with which they have such conflict. That is why we first look for flexibility in a woman's beliefs about abortion to see whether she is able to include herself within the realm of acceptable, understandable, or forgivable abortions. If not, we can gently explore the possibility of flexibility in her decision.

Exercise 5.4

This is an exercise that you can do alone. After you finish, you can compare your findings with a coworker. This exercise will help you to collect phrases that correspond to the different skills within our framework. Use case examples 5.1–5.6 from this chapter for this exercise. Compile some examples where the counselor:

1. Validates and normalizes
2. Seeks understanding of a *feeling*
3. Asks about the *origin* of a feeling
4. Seeks understanding of a *belief*
5. Asks about the *origin* of a belief

Challenging Cases

Talking to angry people is not necessarily a pleasant task! If you are up to the challenge, your mantra is the same as always: validate and seek understanding of the patient's feelings and her beliefs. Be open to learning about her experience. If she becomes defensive at your questioning, validate that you are picking up on her anger, but explain the reasons for your questions. Your hope is that she can feel your compassion and then feel safe enough to reveal the feelings beneath her anger. Patients who are immersed in anger, hostility, and defensiveness are frequently resisting feelings such as fear, shame, and self-hatred. They may have internalized negative, self-directed beliefs from someone else and learned to think negatively about themselves. By remaining steadfast that abortion is murder and that they are committing murder, these patients support a self-image that is negative yet strong and tough. Their anger attempts to banish any sense of weakness, fear, and vulnerability. It can be difficult for you to penetrate this resistance to feeling vulnerable. Seek understanding of negative feelings before reframing. There is no way that an angry patient is going to pay attention to your attempts to put a positive spin on her situation! Validation is your most important tool for working with anger and hostility. When anger and hostility lessen, some of the negative self-directed emotions come to the surface, and the patient may start to cry. You'll be there to support her and let her know that she's in the right place to work through these feelings so that she can feel more comfortable with her abortion decision.

Case Example 5.7

Counselor: What was it like for you to make the decision to have an abortion?

Patient: It was hard, because I don't believe in abortion, but I have to have one.

Counselor: That must make it hard for you to be here.

Patient: [*Rushed*] Yeah, well, it is, but I need to get this done.

Counselor: I'd like to understand your beliefs better. What have you thought about abortion?

Patient: [*Curtly*] I think it's murder.

Counselor: That word means different things to different people. What does it mean to you?

Patient: Look, I have to do this. I am committing murder, and that's what I believe. I keep telling you that and you keep asking me these stupid questions. I want to have an abortion!

Counselor: I can tell that you're frustrated, but my questions are part of the counseling. This clinic is not here to help people commit murder. You are basically asking our physician to participate with you in committing murder. That would make her uncomfortable.

Patient: I don't give a shit how she feels. I'm paying you guys to do this.

Counselor: Well, I care about her, and although you probably don't believe me, I care about you, too, and how you are going to feel after having an abortion.

Patient: I'll be fine. Can we just move on?

Counselor: What got in the way of you continuing this pregnancy?

Patient: I can't have this fucking baby! Don't you get that? I've got no money, I'm alone, and I've got no job. Nobody is there for me!

Counselor: [*Quietly and calmly*] I didn't know that, and I'm sorry to hear that. Things sound really bad for you. You've probably been carrying all this around by yourself with no one to help you. It's not fair that you have had to suffer this way.

Patient: [*Starting to cry*] I've got nobody! Everyone has abandoned me! There's no one who gives a shit about me or my problems.

The patient broke through her anger to let other feelings arise. You may be tempted to take the patient's hostility personally and want to punish her for being rude, hostile, and mean. You may want to turn your back on the now-tearful patient and let her suffer in her emergent feelings. *Do the exact opposite.* Support her and validate her with all of your might. It is a sign of strength, skill, and maturity when a counselor can empathize with a person who was verbally abusive just a few moments before. The wise counselor recognizes that the patient has bravely accessed difficult feelings. Experience teaches that beneath a person's rudeness and hostility are often vulnerability, sadness, grief and loss, and guilt. Here is the person that you were looking for at the beginning of the conversation.

Now proceed with her as you would with any kind of emotional conflict. Acknowledge her dilemma and validate her feelings. Tell her that she is not alone. Offer her information and referrals for emotional healing after the abortion. Talk to her about ways to reframe her decision. Finally, ask her whether there is anything you can do to make her visit better:

Counselor: I care about you. If you need to have this abortion, we are going to take good care of you. Even though we know you don't want to be here, we are going to do everything we can to make your visit here better.

Patient: [*Takes tissues*] Okay.

Counselor: You know, some women have feelings underneath their decision to have an abortion that are hard to feel. Sometimes that is sadness, guilt, loss, or shame. Are you feeling any of these?

Although I am partial to open-ended questions, when patients are really raw and vulnerable I sometimes provide them with a list of feelings so that it doesn't seem like I am trying to overprobe their minds. When I provide examples, I am also motivated by a secondary goal of both normalizing and assessing at the same time. If I tell her that other women feel these feelings, then she doesn't have to worry that something that she says will seem abnormal. On the other hand, you could make the argument that if I provide a list, then she might feel unable to offer a feeling that wasn't included. Explore using both techniques to see which one works better for you.

Patient: I feel guilty. I feel like I'm doing something that's wrong. The baby is innocent. I'm not.

Counselor: Let's go back to your reasons for having the abortion. You pretty much described a situation where you had no support and no one to help you. To me, that doesn't seem like an easy situation. It would probably be a hard situation for having a baby. Am I right?

Patient: Yeah.

Counselor: Let me tell you what I'm getting at. You have reasons for needing to have an abortion. Those are valid reasons. You know why they are valid? It is because they are *your* reasons. *You* are the person who is living your life. You are the *only person* who can know what you need to do. No one else can tell you how to live your life. I trust you on that, and I think that other people should too, even if they aren't showing it right now.

Patient: [*Listening*]

Counselor: So what I am getting at is a different way to look at your decision. You are making a decision based on compassion and mercy, both for yourself and for the baby. Sometimes it's not the right time to have a baby because the woman would suffer or because the baby would suffer. At this clinic, we believe that you are making a *moral* decision. You are trying to prevent suffering. You're doing the best that you can based on where you are with your life.

At this point most women are with you even if they were cursing at you at the beginning. They are nodding their heads and letting some compassion for themselves into their hearts. After you are done with your reframe, check in with her.

Counselor: How do you feel about your decision now?

Patient: I feel better about it.

Counselor: Do you feel ready to finish your paperwork?

Patient: Yes.

Counselor: How do you feel toward yourself?

Patient: I feel better.

Counselor: That's good. It's okay to forgive yourself. It's okay to love yourself, too.

None of us wants to feel vulnerable. Soften your inquiries by explaining the motivations behind your questions. Depending on your clinic's policy, inform the patient of the reasons for your questions. Some clinics let the patient know that their providers do not feel comfortable when patients believe they are committing murder (and are asking providers to conspire to commit murder with them). This can be a way for patients to gain some perspective on the impact of their behavior on others. Even if your clinic will provide abortions for anti-abortion women without requiring any transformation to take place in counseling, it is still beneficial to promote accountability in what patients say to and about others. There are few contexts in our society where abusive and threatening behavior is tolerated without question and service is rendered. Exceptions exist where individuals lack competence. It behooves us as a community to consider the bearing of extreme, negative patient behavior on other patients, on staff, and on the patients themselves. Corrective and ameliorative actions go a long way to making our working environments feel safer and saner.

Case Example 5.8

Counselor: So what was it like for you to make the decision to come here today?

Patient: It was really hard.

Counselor: What made it hard?

Patient: I don't believe in abortion.

Counselor: Can you say more about your beliefs?

Patient: [*Curtly*] I just believe that it's wrong. It's murder. But I'm stuck. I have to have an abortion.

Counselor: I can see why the decision was so hard.

Patient: [*Rudely*] Yeah, well I just need to get it done, so can we finish this up?

At this point, there are several avenues of discussion that the counselor could open up. Because the patient is rushing the counselor, she will need to let her know why she is continuing to ask questions. Depending on your clinic's policy, you may want to add a statement that you are required to talk further with people to understand their use of the word *murder*. Sometimes, a counselor may decide to switch gears and turn to another topic of discussion to try to gain rapport and then come back to seek understanding of the patient's beliefs later. If things are going nowhere, you may need to inform the patient about the clinic's policy regarding moral conflict. Ideally, you can do so in a way that builds empathy for the provider.

Counselor: We are going to finish, but I want to ask you about something you said about abortion being murder. Can you say more about what you mean by that?

Once you and the patient are talking about her use of the word *murder*, you may need to present her with a couple of examples to find out how closely her use of the term matches with definitions of murder. What you are trying to find out is whether she feels that abortion is the same thing as, for example, killing a newborn baby. If someone literally believes that she is committing murder, it's not likely that she will fare well emotionally after the abortion. When I am working with patients with extreme moral conflict, I also have another motivation. I am not interested in allowing women to come to the clinic and talk about abortion as murder, be rude and abusive toward staff, and then demand service. My job is to protect the providers, the clinic, and my coworkers from this kind of abuse and exposure to litigation. I want women to understand the full import of their use of this kind of language; we take them seriously and hold them accountable.

Counselor: Do you think it is the same thing as killing a newborn baby?

Patient: Yes, I do.

Counselor: So for you, having an abortion today would be the same thing as if you took a pillow and smothered a baby.

Patient: Yes.

Counselor: Well, a couple of things come to mind for me. You are equating abortion with murder in the way that most people think about murder as a crime that is punishable by law. If that is the case for you, how do you think you'll feel afterward?

Patient: I'm going to feel like crap, but it's what I have to do. I'll deal with it.

Counselor: How will you deal with it?

Patient: I just will! Can't you leave me alone?

Counselor: Here's what I see from my perspective. You are saying that for you, to have this abortion would be like murdering a newborn baby. At the same time, it's something that you just have to do. I'm worried about how you are going to feel afterward because I can't imagine that someone who commits murder is going to go home afterward and just be able to "deal with it."

Patient: I'll be fine! I just need to get this over with!

Counselor: Well, let me explain where I'm coming from. When people use the word *murder*, I have to ask them about it. At this clinic, we're concerned about how well women can cope after feeling like they have committed murder.

Patient: [*Frustrated*] This is so fucking crazy!

Counselor: You may feel that it's crazy. Let's take a moment to try this again. Look, you don't know me from a hole in the wall. I don't know you. I can tell that you are angry, frustrated, and would rather be just about anywhere else on this earth besides this clinic. Am I right?

Patient: You better fucking believe it!

Counselor: Okay, good. I'm getting an understanding of where you are at. Think with me here just a minute. Are you at all curious as to why I work here?

Patient: No, not really.

Counselor: [*With humor*] You're not at all curious as to why I work here and persist in asking you these annoying questions despite the fact that you are yelling at me?

Patient: [*Reluctantly smiles*]

Counselor: Surely you don't think you're the first person ever to be pissed off here, right?

Patient: No, I'm sure everyone is pissed. You guys make us wait around forever!

Counselor: [*Laughs*] Not everyone is as pissed off as you are, but I have talked to women who are really angry. The point is that I care about how you feel now and how you will feel later. You clearly feel like you are stuck between a rock and a hard place. It seems like someone who dislikes abortion as much as you do would never come here, so you must be in a really tough situation. What is going on for you?

This counselor showed early on that she was taking the patient's words seriously and communicated her motivations. Once you present the rules and that there's no way around them, the patient's anger will likely surge once more. That is an important moment to validate her anger and then tell her why you care about her. Never minimize the patient's anger. Show her that you are taking it seriously. Of course she's frustrated! You're asking her all these personal questions and questions about abortion, and she hates abortion! Who wouldn't want to avoid such as conversation? It's just that avoidance and denial only work for so long.

Once women realize how seriously you are taking them, they may back down a little and admit exaggeration. Sometimes patients use words like *murder* and *killing* to express anger. Anger can be a cover for tremendous disappointment in a relationship; a pregnancy can be the catalyst for this discovery. In the case above, the counselor used some self-deprecating humor. Remember, if you can validate her anger, frustration, boredom, or irritation, it has less power to consume you *and* her. If you can gain rapport by aligning yourself with her situation, then you are skillfully doing so in one of the most challenging contexts.

Case Example 5.9

In this example, the counselor refers to clinic policy to help the patient understand the motivation behind her questions. She also attempts to build empathy for the provider and encourages the patient to reflect on how her feelings and statements do not upset only the provider, but other staff within the clinic.

Patient: I think abortion is murder.

Counselor: Do you think it is the same thing as killing a newborn baby?

Patient: Yes, I do.

Counselor: So for you, having an abortion today would be the same thing as if you took a pillow and smothered a baby.

Patient: Yes.

Counselor: What about if you took out a gun and shot me, right here in the clinic? For you, is abortion the same thing as that?

Patient: Yes. It's murder.

Counselor: I can imagine that it must be hard for you to be here. I can also imagine that it's not going to be very easy for you afterward.

Patient: [*Irritated*] Well, I just need to get this done. You people need to move faster here!

Counselor: Well, there are a couple of things that I need to ask you. How do you imagine that the doctor will feel once I tell her that for you, this abortion is the same thing as killing a newborn baby or taking out a gun and shooting her?

Patient: [*Nonchalantly*] I don't know.

Counselor: I can tell you that she's going to be very concerned. I'm not sure that it is fair for you to ask her to participate in committing murder with you, or *for* you. It's important to think about how that might make *her* feel.

Patient: [*Silent*]

Counselor: I can tell you that it would make her feel terrible. She works here because she believes that she is helping women who are in really tough situations who have decided that abortion is the best decision that they can make at this time in their lives.

Patient: [*Silent*]

Counselor: I'm imagining that you hadn't thought about it this way, and that your intention wasn't to make our doctor feel uncomfortable. Am I right?

Patient: [*Nods*] Yes.

Counselor: The other thing is that it is hard for me to imagine that it would be very easy for you to commit murder and then go about your life. I'm worried about you and how you'll do afterward.

Patient: [*Silent*]

Counselor: [*Gently*] What's been going on for you?

Allow the patient to sit with this for a moment. The point is not to punish her. The point is to show her that she is accountable for her behavior in the clinic, including her language. It is also to show her the power of her language and to give her the opportunity to really think about what she means by what she says. You'll want to give her a space to talk about the feelings that underlie her choice of words.

Case Example 5.10

If you are encountering hostility, rudeness, or silence, let the patient know the motivation behind your questions. Let her know that your clinic does not tolerate disrespectful communication. Under no circumstances should any clinic tolerate threatening behavior or physical assault from a patient. If you have a policy about moral conflict, let the patient know why you need to get a better understanding of her decision. In case example 5.10, the counselor explains clinic policy while at the same time underlining the clinic's concern for the patient's well-being. It is an example of an extreme situation because the counselor experiences some verbal abuse but eventually establishes rapport with the patient. You are unlikely to ever encounter a counseling moment this extreme. Nevertheless, it is imperative that clinic staff have an opportunity to discuss their feelings and thoughts surrounding how they wish to work with these situations in a unified manner. Feeling safe and supported is paramount to a healthy working environment.

Patient: You know what? I don't feel like talking to you about this!

Counselor: I get that you don't feel like talking. I can imagine that this whole thing has not been a pleasant experience for you. Let me tell you why I am asking you these questions. It is our clinic policy to try to understand what people mean when they use words like *murder*.

Patient: I don't give a shit what your clinic policy is! I want to get this over with.

Counselor: Talking to me is part of the process of getting your abortion. Talking to the doctor is part of it, too. We can't go forward without talking about this. Maybe you and I got off to a bad start. Do you want to take five minutes and then I'll meet you back here and we can try again?

Patient: Screw you lady! This is bullshit!

Counselor: One thing that's not okay here is disrespectful communication. There is another clinic in town that could help you, and maybe you'd be more comfortable there. You are welcome to stay here if you agree to respectful communication. But as long as we continue on this way, we won't provide care for you today.

When patients are so hostile and abusive that you are concerned for your safety, you need to get your supervisor. As long as I feel safe, I usually will try one more summary statement to persuade the patient to see things from my point of view. If she doesn't respond positively, I will ask her to leave.

Counselor: Look, I am reading loud and clear that you are angry with me for asking these questions. But take a moment to think about it from my point of view and the clinic's point of view. You have come into our workplace, demanded that we provide you with a service, and then called what we do here "murder."

Now that I have her attention, I will go back—one more time—and attempt to reach her and what is really going on beneath her anger and hostility.

Counselor: I can imagine that there is a lot going on for you and that you are in a tough situation. But truly, I don't even know anything about you yet. It's worth trying to make this a better experience for you. You are worth it. Let's start again and communicate respectfully with one another. What do you say?

Patient: [*Quietly but firmly*] Okay.

Counselor: I know that you're not thrilled to be here. Maybe you are feeling sick, nauseated, and exhausted. Maybe you've been trying to get an abortion for a long time. You may have used your last dollar just to get here today. I don't know your particulars because we have barely begun talking to each other. But I'm sure that things haven't been completely great. Am I right?

Patient: [*Irritated*] Yes.

Counselor: [*Gently*] What's been going on for you?

Patient: [*Frustrated*] You know, I really don't want to talk to you about this.

Counselor: What is your biggest concern about talking to me?

Patient: Because it's none of your business!

Counselor: Part of it actually *is* my business. Let me explain. There are people who come to abortion clinics demanding an abortion yet believe that abortion is murder or should be illegal. Afterward, some of those same women are very upset. They have a lot of regret. Then they decide that the clinic is responsible for their suffering and should have prevented them from having an abortion. In this clinic, our policy is that we talk to patients in order to understand where they are coming from. Sometimes, we ask them to reschedule their appointment.

Patient: But I'm paying for this! You have to give me an abortion!

Counselor: Actually, we don't. We have the same rights to refuse service as any other organization.

Patient: This is ridiculous!

Counselor: [*Matter-of-factly*] You can go to another clinic, but there's a chance that they will ask the same questions. Of course, you can answer differently and lead them to believe that you are fine with your decision. So you're free to leave here and go elsewhere. I'm not asking you these questions to make you angry. This is our policy because we know that women who feel the way that you do don't cope well after their abortion. Look at it logically: how could you expect a woman who believes that she is committing murder to feel fine afterward?

Patient: [*Silent*]

Counselor: Can you see what I'm saying, even a little bit?

Patient: [*Reluctantly*] I suppose.

Counselor: Let's see whether you and I can start over. [*Long pause*] Who came with you today?

Patient: No one.

Counselor: Is there anyone who knows that you are pregnant?

Patient: The father, he knows.

Counselor: What did he say when you told him?

Patient: He didn't say anything except for "You'd better get rid of it," and then I haven't seen him since.

Counselor: I'm sorry about that.

Patient: He's a jerk and that's typical for him.

Counselor: How did you feel when he said that?

Patient: Shitty.

Counselor: Was that the beginning of things being bad for you?

Patient: Oh yeah. Things have been nothing but bad since I got pregnant.

Counselor: What's been going on?

After a great deal of persistence, the counselor succeeded in gaining some rapport with the patient and actually steered things back to the patient's feelings. But before that, she held her ground knowing that the clinic would back her if she asked this patient to leave. She also asked the patient to see it from the provider's perspective, the clinic's perspective, and the perspective of an outsider: How would it not warrant proceeding with caution when a woman is unwavering in her beliefs that abortion is murder? After discussing the patient's struggles and empathizing with her, the counselor can go back to exploring her beliefs about abortion. I have had interactions such as these; fortunately, they were few and far between. Even the few times that things were this bad, most patients warmed to staff eventually. I do require that the patient acknowledge her behavior and apologize if she swore at a staff member or called her names. But I always empathize with the patient for what must have been going on for her to behave in such a manner.

FINAL THOUGHTS

Counseling patients with moral conflict can be tremendously challenging. We can become unnerved in the face of patient anger and flummoxed by the juxtaposition of anti-abortion sentiment and decision certainty. The same tools that we use for working with emotional conflict can help us work with moral conflict. We must treat anger the same way that we treat sadness—validate it and seek to understand it and where it is coming from. Repeat the exercises and rehearse the dialogue until you find your own voice and your own style. It takes a long time for this kind of work to feel natural. It takes practice. You'll learn more from your mistakes than from your successes. Don't give up!

Moral conflict raises difficult issues in our community around our obligations and responsibilities toward women seeking abortion who at the same time hold extreme, negative opinions about abortion. Get clarity on your personal values and your clinic's policies. Clinic discussions that lead to the creation of policies around how to work with angry, abusive, and anti-abortion patients give staff a feeling of safety, support, and clear parameters surrounding job expectations. Clinic discussions on this topic also serve to reduce feelings of isolation and confusion that can lead to staff burnout and resentment toward patients. It helps to take on these challenges with a unified voice. As social scientists unravel the emotional consequences of having abortions in the context of moral conflict, we will feel better informed about how to proceed in these circumstances. In the meantime, we can use the data that we have on factors that are associated with suboptimal coping after an abortion. We also are guided by our values and beliefs as humanistic, patient-centered providers. Our humanistic perspective guides our work not only with our patients but also with one another. As we care for our patients, we must also care for ourselves.

Chapter Six

Decision Counseling
for Ambivalence

Not every woman who comes to an abortion clinic is sure that she wants to have an abortion. While this is a small minority of patients, it's an important one. For some, making the appointment on the phone and then "no-showing" is part of the decision-making process. For others, making the trip to the clinic, getting checked in, and sitting in the waiting room is an important component as well. At the clinic, the counseling session may be the first safe space where a woman has the opportunity to really think about her decision away from the pressures and judgments of others. Having the space to verbalize ambivalence and conflicted feelings can help her reach resolution about having an abortion. Or it could be the moment where she realizes that it would be best for her to reschedule her appointment and take more time to think about what she wants to do.

The different ways that we approach ambivalence are revelatory of our feelings about ambivalence, its place in the abortion clinic, and our role in guiding patients toward resolution. Some patients have spent hours, days, or weeks making the decision prior to coming to the clinic and are still unsure about what to do. For others, their decision was clear from the moment that they discovered they were pregnant. Others fall somewhere in between. Those who are not sure about their decision will, in general, reveal their ambivalence when asked about what it was like for them to make the decision to have an abortion. Clinics differ in their policies as to whether (and how) to assess ambivalence and what (if anything) to do about it once it is discovered. This chapter will provide you with the skills to engage patients in conversations about their ambivalence and exercises to uncover your feelings and beliefs about this issue.

Sometimes, our desire to avoid conversations about patient ambivalence is revelatory of our insecurity and discomfort about how to work with it.

This kind of discomfort is completely understandable. Ambivalence can be intimidating. How can we help someone who is unsure about what to do? It challenges our assumptions about our patients: Why did she come to her appointment today? This is a valid question! That's why we use what we are thinking and feeling as a conversational guide. It helps us become more attuned, more skilled, and more nimble. When we can figure out what pushes our buttons or makes us the most confused, we can tune in to our feelings to get a stronger read on what is going on with our patient. Use what makes you uncomfortable as an important source of information.

Exercise 6.1

In a quiet space, take a moment to think about how you feel when patients present with ambivalence. Write your thoughts in your counseling journal.

1. What feelings come up for you? Where are the feelings coming from?
2. Take it one step further: Think about how ambivalence is treated in abortion politics. How does the anti-abortion (pro-life) community talk about women's ambivalence about abortion? How does the reproductive justice (pro-choice) community talk about it?
3. Finally, think about your own clinic's view of patient ambivalence: What role, if any, are staff expected to have in helping patients resolve it?

When I ask, "What was it like to make the decision to have an abortion?" the ambivalent patient will sometimes say that it was a hard decision. When I ask, "What made it hard?" she may respond that she has spent a long time trying to decide which way is the right way to go or that she has gone back and forth between continuing the pregnancy and having the abortion. Or she may sometimes just come right out and say, "I'm actually not sure if this is what I want to do."

It is important to note that not all women for whom it was a "hard" decision or who have been going back and forth for a long time are ambivalent. She may be filling you in on how it's been for her over the past few days, weeks, or months. When I ask, "How are you feeling right now about your decision?" she may come back with, "Oh, I'm okay now; it's just that it took me a long time to get clear on what was best." In that case, I take a moment to validate her process and commend her on having taken the time to do the work of decision making. But if the patient says, "Yeah, I'm actually still as unsure as I was three weeks ago," then I know that I am embarking on a conversation about ambivalence.

Research shows women's reasons for having abortions can be grouped into two broad categories: a desire to be able to care for children that they already have and a desire to be prepared to care for children that they may have in the future (Finer et al. 2005). A woman may disclose that her family is complete; she may want another child in the future but now is not the right time due to financial or relationship issues; or she may never want children. Most women who come to an abortion clinic are not ambivalent. They have weighed the pros and cons of each option and decided that abortion is the best decision for them, given their life circumstances. The ambivalent patient, however, is *stuck*. She may be experiencing a conflict between her beliefs and her planned behavior. She may be unable to access her own desire among the sea of desires and judgments of others.

For some ambivalent patients, the decision is complicated because the reasons against one option do not lead to an obvious and smooth election of another option. The bumper sticker that states, "Against abortion? Don't have one!" may be a satisfying retort but is too simple of a framework for understanding decision conflict on an individual level. Some of our patients do state that they are against abortion. They may also insist that there's no way that they can continue the pregnancy. Your job is to find out *how much* against abortion the patient really is, *how* impossible it would be to continue the pregnancy, and *whether* she would consider adoption. Then, you can see whether she can introduce some flexibility into her beliefs or into her decision. The possibility of flexibility in her beliefs or decision can be found in the conversation between counselor and patient. Remember that *the patient has the answer* to her dilemma.

Counseling for ambivalence is different from counseling for emotional, spiritual, and moral conflict in that it requires some additional steps. In counseling for conflict, the patient is often sure that abortion is the best option, but she is struggling with feelings and thoughts that she has about abortion or about herself. Ambivalent patients may have emotional, spiritual, or moral conflict with abortion, but they are unsure as to which pregnancy option is the better one for them. Ambivalence counseling also is different from options counseling in that options counseling involves a patient who is in an exploratory stage—she is seeking information about her options; she has not yet begun to align herself with one decision. A patient who is ambivalent has made an appointment for an abortion, yet she is unable to go through with it. She made movement toward a decision but is unable to commit.

WHAT IS AMBIVALENCE?

Merriam-Webster Online defines ambivalence in three ways: first, as "simultaneous and contradictory attitudes or feelings (as attraction and repulsion) toward an object, person, or action." Second, it is seen as "a continual fluctuation (as between one thing and its opposite)." Finally, ambivalence can be "uncertainty as to which approach to follow." In the context of decision making, this leads to a feeling of being stuck in the process of decision making because a case can be made for more than one alternative. The source of a patient's conflict with abortion can be emotional, spiritual, or moral. The source of a patient's conflict over parenting can be an abusive or absent partner, financial issues, a lack of readiness to be a parent, or a lack of support. The source of a patient's conflict over adoption can be guilt, grief, and loss. The ambivalent patient is simultaneously experiencing emotions about abortion and emotions about continuing the pregnancy that are in conflict with one another and are impeding her ability to make a decision.

Here are examples of *indirect* behaviors that can indicate ambivalence:

- The patient is quiet or makes little eye contact.
- The patient rushes the counselor.
- The patient has an aggressive or demanding parent or partner who wants to be with her at all times.
- Her parent or partner made her appointment.
- She is taking prenatal vitamins.
- She has rescheduled her appointment several times.

Here are some examples of statements from patients that are *direct* indications of ambivalence:

- I'm not sure what I want to do.
- I still don't know whether this is the best decision for me.
- I feel torn.
- Can I have the laminaria removed if I change my mind?
- If I have to wait any longer, I might not go through with it.

Ambivalent patients are torn over which option is best and which decision will produce the fewest of the least desirable outcomes. They may be struggling to access their true desires. They may feel overwhelmed by the desires and demands of others concerning what they "should" do. An ambivalent patient may state that she *wants* to continue the pregnancy but feels she has many reasons to have an abortion. An ambivalent patient may be opposed to abortion for herself but concerned about continuing the pregnancy because her male partner is abusive and controlling. At the emotional core of many cases of ambivalence is a conflict between the head (what one thinks is the best decision) and the heart (one's emotions and attachments) (Kimport

2010). Unable to fully trust in herself, a woman paralyzed by ambivalence cannot sit with the idea that she herself is making the decision to end a pregnancy. She may want fate to intervene—such as an ultrasound indicating that she is too far along to have the abortion or evidence that she is miscarrying or that there is "something wrong with the baby." Patients often can speak explicitly about how they wish an act of fate could be "responsible" for making the decision.

Sometimes patients get a lot of relief from hearing that they are not the only person who has felt this way. This is part of normalizing and validating. The event of pregnancy has brought them down a road. At the end of the road there is a fork—one way is continuing the pregnancy, and the other way is having an abortion. One way must be chosen. For some women, *neither* path is desirable or feels like a good decision, but one way must eventually emerge as the *better* of the two. This metaphor can provide patients with some relief from relentless guilt over having an abortion because it gives them permission to acknowledge that continuing the pregnancy would not be without problems either.

APPROACH AND FRAMEWORK

Let's take a moment to review the three components of our *approach* in the context of counseling for ambivalence:

1. Listen.
2. Do not assume!
3. Self-reflect.

Be an active, engaged listener. This communicates interest and respect. Be curious about and genuinely concerned with the patient's well-being. If you are bored, afraid, distant, stiff, or judgmental when talking to a patient on the telephone or in person, she will instantly pick up on that and give it right back to you! You reap what you sow: the seeds that you plant in your approach to your patient determine what will grow between you. If you give respect and compassion, usually you will get it back. If you are interested in learning more about the patient, she will be more willing to share.

Do not make assumptions about which pregnancy option is better for your patient. Be curious and genuinely explore different possibilities. Listen for possibilities, put one forward, and ask your patient to dwell in that space. It is easy for us to become stuck in our assumptions—that everyone coming to an abortion clinic wants an abortion, that hardly anyone considers adoption, or that there's no way the patient could continue the pregnancy. Counseling for ambivalence challenges our habitual mode of being pulled around by our assumptions. You are not responsible for setting the agenda for the conversation. The patient's story is the path of your conversation. Her feelings, beliefs, and values will determine her decision. Use what you are thinking and feeling to guide your questions and comments. Do a self-assessment—what about ambivalence is difficult for you? What feelings and concerns are hardest for you to talk about? In what circumstances are you biased against a patient continuing the pregnancy? How do you feel about adoption? Self-reflection is a first step toward allowing your weaknesses to become your strengths.

The framework that we have used for counseling for the three types of conflict is also used when counseling for ambivalence (see box 6.1). The unique aspect of ambivalence counseling is an additional skill that we will utilize at level 3. The work of reframing includes the technique of listen—put forward—dwell. The key issue with ambivalence is that the patient is stuck—perhaps her conflict with abortion is significant and her perceived roadblocks to continuing the pregnancy seem insurmountable. Your goal as her facilitator and guide will be to help her discover flexibility in her beliefs or flexibility in her decision. One of these positions must become more flexible in order for her to resolve her ambivalence. As we will see in the case examples, listen—put forward—dwell is a technique that reflects back to the patient *her own* perspective of which options are realistic and acceptable in order to loosen ambivalence and open the path toward a decision.

Box 6.1. Framework

Level 1: Validate and normalize.
Level 2: Seek understanding.
Level 3: Reframe.

LEVEL 1: VALIDATE AND NORMALIZE

As we move through different counseling scenarios, I will give examples of counseling on each of the three levels in our framework. Validation and normalization are important ways to let the patient know that you have noticed her ambivalence. She may come right out and say that she is not sure about the decision, or she may be more stoic and reticent. Recognize the ambivalence, and verbalize it for both of you to reflect on. Remind your patient that you are here to help her sort through her thoughts and feelings. If she seems distressed by her ambivalence, reinforce that this is why you are here and that you have helped other women work through these issues. Let her know that she is in the right place to think about her decision.

LEVEL 2: SEEK UNDERSTANDING

As always, seek understanding of feelings that are expressed in your patient's language or in her bodily comportment. If she is crying, witness her tears and give her a space to cry. Ask her to say more about her feelings and where they are coming from. By exploring her feelings, you are trying to discover the origin of the conflict with abortion. Is it emotional, spiritual, or moral? You'll also want to explore any beliefs that are at the core of her conflict with abortion, adoption, and parenting. Be curious and interested to learn more about these beliefs. Where did they come from? Are there exceptions? The story, the certainty scale, and tracking her pros and cons on the six dimensions of pregnancy decision making are the techniques that you can use to seek understanding.

The Patient's Story

Conversations about ambivalence are guided by the patient's narrative of what has taken place in her life from the moment she found out she was pregnant up to the moment she is talking to you at the clinic. You are listening for her thoughts and feelings regarding different pregnancy options (abortion, adoption, and parenting) and how those have changed or not changed over the course of time leading up to your counseling session. As you listen to her story, you will collect data on her arguments for and against each of the three pregnancy options. Because there are three options and reasons for and against each, you'll be collecting data on six dimensions of pregnancy decision making (see figure 6.1). Remember that reasons *against* the abortion are not necessarily the same thing as reasons *for* continuing the pregnancy. Ask questions that will help you better understand why the patient feels adoption is impossible or continuing the pregnancy is desirable. Don't assume or try to guess what she thinks or feels about each option—ask her. As you gain a better understanding of her reasons pro and con, listen for places where you can ask her to dwell with different possibilities.

The patient's story is an invaluable tool when patients are having trouble sorting through or accessing their feelings. Sometimes people are so confused about what they are thinking and feeling that it is easier to focus on recounting events that led up to today. There is not a specific set of rules on how she should tell her story. This is a space for her to talk and for you to listen. The

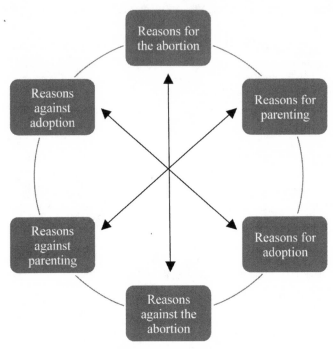

Figure 6.1. Six Dimensions of Pregnancy Decision Making

story is the *engine* behind the entire conversation. The patient will lead you down the path that she has taken to get to the clinic. The path is the movement of time toward the future. The places of conflict, doubt, and second thoughts are detours off that path. These detours signify moments where she has been pulled by other people's feelings or her own feelings about what she *should* do or which is the *right* decision.

The Certainty Scale

A great way to get perspective on a patient's ambivalence is to take a measurement of her level of certainty. This can be done in conjunction with asking her to tell her story or in place of it. Use the scale to get a reading on the patient's level of certainty as soon as you suspect ambivalence; repeat the scale later in the conversation to see whether there has been any change.

Patient: I had such a hard time making this decision. I went back and forth a lot before coming here today.

Counselor: That's true for a lot of women. I'm glad you've shared that with me. I'd like to get an idea of how you're feeling today. On a scale from one to ten, if one is being sure that continuing the pregnancy is the best decision and ten is being sure that abortion is the best decision, where are you now?

Where ambivalence ends and certainty begins on this scale is a matter of opinion. I use seven or eight or greater as an indicator of sufficient certainty to be able to consent to the abortion. If a patient states that she is a seven, eight, or nine, I will ask her what is keeping her from being a ten, but I won't require her to get there. It is okay to still have feelings, both current and anticipated, that keep people from being 100 percent certain. In life, many important decisions are made without 100 percent certainty, such as whether or whom to marry, whether to get a divorce, which school to attend, or which job to take. The most important thing is that we are able to understand our reasons for making the decision and remember that it was the best one we could have made at that time in our lives.

When patients are ambivalent, they will often be at five or six. I reflect back my interpretation of her number, just to be sure I'm not assuming that my understanding of the scale is the same as hers. I might say, "So you're at a five. You're really unsure about which way you want to go." Then I look for her response to see whether we are in agreement.

Find out whether she has a different number for her "head" and for her "heart" (see case example 6.4, later in this chapter). That will help to separate what she *thinks* is the best decision from how she *feels* about the decision, that is, her sadness, guilt, and grief. Sometimes people have a much higher number for their head than for their heart. Check in with your patient to see whether she knows why there is such a big difference between her head and her heart. Typically it is because she feels that abortion is best, given her life circumstances, but she also feels very conflicted about it emotionally, spiritually, or morally. Determine the source of the conflict by asking her what is getting in the way of her being a ten.

Counselor: Okay, you're at a seven—more of you wants to have the abortion. What's keeping you from being a ten?

Patient: I feel guilty.

Counselor: Do you have a sense of where your guilt is coming from?

Seek understanding of the meaning of her feelings and their origins. For example, when a patient discloses feelings of guilt, I want to figure out whether she feels guilty because she thinks abortion is selfish, feels irresponsible for not using birth control or having a birth control failure, worries that God will not forgive her, or wants an abortion and her partner does not. In all these circumstances, the *feeling* of guilt is attached to different *contexts*. I want to understand the context in which the feeling of guilt occurs to see whether I can offer a different way of thinking about abortion. That's the key to reframing. You aren't telling the patient not to feel her feelings—on the contrary. You are introducing a possibility of *thinking* about them in a different way. In summary, there are times when I use only the certainty scale (including head versus. heart) and never explicitly ask the patient to tell her story. In these cases, I feel like I get all my information from her answer to "What's keeping you from being a ten?" There are other times when I ask her to tell her story and never use the certainty scale. There's no right or wrong way.

LEVEL 3: REFRAME

Exploring feelings and beliefs prepares you to attempt a reframe of the abortion decision. If your patient is feeling guilt, ask her where her guilt is coming from. Understanding the source of her guilt is a necessary step in preparing to reframe. If her guilt is coming from her understanding of fetal development, fetal pain, or how the procedure is performed, you can reframe by providing her with correct medical information. You may also discover that she has incomplete information about adoption law or her confidentiality rights. These concerns often are alleviated with accurate information. If her guilt is coming from a concern about what God thinks about her, then you've discovered that her conflict is spiritual in origin. Enter into a conversation around spiritual conflict, and seek understanding of her beliefs and what is getting in the way of her feeling included in any positive beliefs. Then use her own beliefs to reframe her view of herself and the abortion.

The overarching aim when engaging in ambivalence counseling is to collaboratively discover flexibility in the patient's beliefs or flexibility in the patient's decision. Listen—put forward—dwell and reframing are the techniques that you will use to uncover this flexibility. What's unique about the ambivalent patient is that the first attempt at reframing often doesn't work. That isn't to say that it doesn't help, but rather that it doesn't always bring resolution. She may still feel pulled toward another option. She may be listening intently to what you are saying but after a moment of silence will exclaim, "I still don't know what to do!" When reframing an option that she is drawn to does not succeed in loosening her ambivalence, you'll turn to an exploration and reframing of each of her other options. If she rejects these, you'll return to seeking flexibility in her beliefs about the option that she is drawn to through another reframe.

Reframing

At level 3, the counselor offers the patient a different way to think about *herself* and her *decision*. For example, the patient may have been exposed to anti-abortion propaganda that has created a lot of fear about the abortion; she could be worried about how the procedure is performed or whether she'll become infertile afterward. She may have heard that an abortion is performed using "knives" and "hooks" to "cut the baby out." She may think that her twenty-two-week (or nine-week) fetus is the same size as a full-term, newborn baby. Providing accurate medical information on the following topics produces relief and can resolve ambivalence:

- The safety of abortion
- That abortion does not affect fertility
- The technique of electric vacuum aspiration and manual vacuum aspiration
- The size of the embryo or fetus
- The amount of cervical dilation needed for D&E versus a vaginal delivery
- The fetus's capacity to feel pain

You also may discover that the source of a patient's ambivalence is misinformation about facts, laws, and rights about adoption. Countering misinformation about adoption requires that the counselor research the laws of her state. Contact open adoption agencies in your area to establish a referral connection. Screen potential adoption agency partners by asking them whether they are "pro-choice" and how they put that philosophy into practice. You are looking for an agency that

- provides options counseling and refers patients for abortion services when that is what the patient prefers.
- has a philosophy that recognizes abortion and adoption as morally equivalent choices.
- prioritizes the experience and well-being of the birth mother.

The Adoption Access Network is a network of adoption agencies in the United States that adhere to these values. Information is available on the website http://www.adoptionaccessnetwork.org/. Educate yourself on the availability of open adoption in your state, paternal rights, minors' rights to place a child for adoption, and temporary foster care or kin adoption options. When a patient's ambivalence originates in emotional, spiritual, or moral conflict regarding abortion, use what you've learned in previous chapters to seek understanding and offer a reframe.

Case Example 6.1

Patient: Mostly what I've been feeling is guilt.

Counselor: Can you put your finger on where your guilt is coming from?

Patient: Well, I just feel like having this abortion is selfish. I feel so selfish.

Counselor: Can you say more about that?

Patient: It seems selfish to have the abortion, doing something that *I* want and not caring about the baby.

Counselor: Do you know where that idea is coming from?

Patient: It just seems like something that a mother isn't supposed to do.

Counselor: I've heard other women say similar things. When I look closely at your situation, I see a woman doing her best to take care of three small children with very little help from others. You've said that your reasons for having an abortion are so that you can better take care of the children that you have. That doesn't seem selfish. That seems like a caring, selfless decision. What if you thought about it that way?

Patient: Thank you for saying that. I've never heard it put that way before.

The source of guilt can be emotional conflict (I'm worried that the baby will feel pain), spiritual conflict (Will God forgive me?), or moral conflict (I feel like I'm killing my baby). You'll want to explore those statements on a deeper level to allow for the possibility of flexibility in the patient's spiritual beliefs (If you believe God is a loving God and that he forgives, why wouldn't he forgive you, too?) or moral values (Now that I have explained more about the embryo, does having an abortion seem like the same thing as killing a newborn baby?). What is unique about the ambivalent patient is that the first attempt at reframing often does not bring resolution. Even if ambivalence persists, the reframe is still an important part of the process.

Listen—Put Forward—Dwell

When using the technique of listen—put forward—dwell (see figure 6.2), you are listening for openings where the patient reveals what would make abortion, adoption, or parenting realistic and acceptable. I call this listening for possibilities. Listening for, putting forward, and dwelling with different possibilities creates a space where the patient can consider options. When you hear something that could make an option possible, ask your patient to dwell there. Start by putting forward the options that *she* has brought up. As a neutral facilitator, you are merely repeating what she has proposed and giving her the opportunity to wonder, "What *if* I did that?" You must set aside

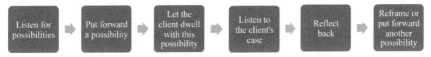

Figure 6.2. Listen—Put Forward—Dwell

any feelings that *you* might have about her options; only she can determine what is best for her. You may need to come back to an option more than once, especially if reframing is not working and her ambivalence persists.

Exercise 6.2

Take another look at the six dimensions of pregnancy decision making in figure 6.1. Read the following possibility statements and pair each one with one of the six dimensions.

- My husband's mother said that she would help us raise the baby.
- Having an abortion would get me away from my abusive partner.
- If my baby could know that I was his birth mother, I would consider adoption.
- There is a teen parenting program at my school. I'd be able to graduate.
- My dad told me that he and his wife would adopt the baby.
- If I have an abortion, I could attend college in the fall on full scholarship.

Possibility statements do not mean that the patient is no longer ambivalent. They merely suggest avenues toward a decision. The real work comes after you hear one of these statements. Together you'll put forward a possibility, look at the pros and cons, and imagine it as reality. It is the patient's responsibility to accept or reject it. Here are some ways to put forward possibilities for the patient to consider:

- What would be *good* about having an abortion? What would *not* be good?
- What *if* you did a kin adoption with your aunt and uncle?
- What would be *good* about having the baby? What would *not* be good?
- What *if* you asked your guidance counselor for help in getting into the teen parent program at school?

Eventually, one decision will emerge as the one that has the most positives and fewest negatives associated with it. It will be the decision that the patient is most willing and able to live with. The more stuck a patient is, the more times you will put forward different possibilities for her consideration.

Listen to the Patient's Case

The patient's case is her argument for or against a pregnancy option and the reasons why it is or isn't realistic and acceptable. Listen to the case that your patient makes so that you understand why it would or would not work. You may need to return to a possibility that she has rejected if she remains adamant that the other options are also impossible. As the patient dwells with and thinks about how she feels about different options, her thoughts and feelings will change. She may reach a moment of clarity. She may strengthen her argument for or against a particular option. At times, it may seem as if she is trying to *talk herself into* a particular option. Reflect back what you observe.

Reflecting Back

Reflecting back is a way of summarizing the pros and cons of a pregnancy option that the patient is considering. It allows the patient to review what she has said and to verify whether you have understood her. When you reflect back, validate her conundrum. Then offer a reframe of an option that she is considering in order to determine whether that changes anything. If it does not, ask her what is getting in the way of accepting the reframe. Put forward another possibility that was previously rejected and ask her to dwell with it. When patients are opposed to parenting or adoption *and* remain inflexible and distressed regarding their negative beliefs about abortion, reengage them in a conversation about parenting or adoption. Remember that when you are putting forward a possibility, *you* don't have an agenda for one option over the other. To be effective, you must remain neutral. Your only goal is to help the patient find the answer within herself and resolve her ambivalence. Sometimes, patients cycle between arguments for and against the same option. An important part of the counselor's job is to keep the patient company through this exploration and reflect back her observations.

Case Example 6.2

Patient: My family really wants me to continue this pregnancy. My mom didn't understand why I was coming to the appointment today. Everyone has so many different opinions about what I should do, and it is really confusing.

Counselor: Let's think about the option of continuing the pregnancy. What would be good about that?

Patient: A big part of me has been really excited about having another baby. I love children. My mom bought all this stuff for a nursery, but I didn't ask her to, and that has really contributed to my confusion.

Counselor: Okay, let's look at the other side. What would be not good about continuing the pregnancy?

Patient: The father of the baby, the abuse, my wanting to get away from him. This is a drama that has been going on for a long time.

Counselor: Let's see whether I have an understanding of what's going on for you. What I hear you saying is that a part of you is very excited about the idea of having another baby because of your love of children. There is another part of you that is very concerned about what it would mean to have a child with the father of this baby.

Patient: That's exactly it.

The Importance of Talking about Continuing the Pregnancy

Bringing up the option of continuing the pregnancy is important because it communicates that you have no investment in your patient having an abortion. It lets her know that you are not there to talk her into having an abortion or that the clinic only wants to make money. You may be the first or one of few people in her life who is supporting her in making the best decision for *herself*, no matter which decision it is. Talking about continuing the pregnancy is also especially helpful in defusing tension in conversations with teens who feel they are being forced to have the abortion by one or both parents. It communicates that you are not the enemy and gives the patient a nonjudgmental, unbiased space in which to think about the reality of parenthood.

Patients who are in the throes of ambivalence may give examples of friends or family who have promised to help take care of the baby. Your patient will have an idea of how authentic those offers for help are and how much she can trust in them. Don't make assumptions about her perceptions of those offers; ask her what it would be like if she seriously considered them. Your job is to pose the question, "What *if* your boyfriend's aunt helped you take care of the baby for the first two years?" "What *if* your dad adopted the baby?" This is the time to bring up options such as kin adoption and temporary foster care to see whether she finds these options realistic and acceptable. Ambivalent patients need to dwell in the possibilities that might make continuing the pregnancy possible.

It is important to keep in mind that patients who are *not* ambivalent sometimes talk about a part of themselves that desires to continue the pregnancy. A woman may state how much she loves children and would like another child, but financial and relationship circumstances are not right. If things were different in her life, she would continue the pregnancy. Support her by validating her love for children and reminding her that she can plan for another pregnancy when the time is right. Remind her that it is because of her love of children and concern for their well-being that she is even considering abortion. Together you can make a plan for rituals or mementos that she can use to symbolize or memorialize her love for the baby. This is a powerful reframing of the abortion decision.

Dwelling in the possibilities of parenting and adoption with a patient challenges the *counselor* to grow and change. It revolutionizes our understanding of our role. By truly living the principle that the patient has the answer, we approach this challenge with openness and curiosity. The first time that one of your patients leaves the clinic to continue the pregnancy or place the baby for adoption is when you begin to appreciate the awesome responsibility of being a guardian of informed consent.

Using Hypothetical Situations

Hypothetical situations are tools that you can use when you and your patient are feeling really stuck.

> *Counselor:* Is there any part of you that wished that during the ultrasound the nurse had discovered that you were too far into your pregnancy to be seen here?
>
> *Patient:* No, I'm glad that I still have the option.
>
> *Counselor:* So it sounds like a part of you did not want the option of having an abortion taken away from you. What is getting in the way of you really owning that and having the abortion?

Here's an example where the patient responds in the opposite way:

> *Counselor:* Is there any part of you that wished that during the ultrasound, the nurse had discovered that you were too far into your pregnancy to be seen here?
>
> *Patient:* Yeah, a part of me was hoping I was too far.
>
> *Counselor:* It sounds like a part of you wants fate to intervene and make the decision for you. What do you think that's about?

Exercise 6.3

Let's examine three ways to use hypothetical situations. Think about each in the context of the fundamental principle that *the patient has the answer*. Write your thoughts in your counseling journal.

> *Counselor A:* I'm hearing that a big part of you wants to continue the pregnancy. Why not just go home today? You can always make another appointment if you change your mind.

Counselor B: What if I made the decision for you and told you that you had to go home today and not have the abortion?

Counselor C: The part of you that wants to continue the pregnancy is making a lot of really good points. I think that it's important for you to pay attention to that part and honor those feelings. I'm thinking that leaving today and thinking about what we've talked about would be beneficial to you in the long run. If you become certain that abortion is the best decision, you can always come back. What do you think about that?

Each of the three counselors in exercise 6.3 puts forward the option of not having the abortion today. Some readers may feel that these proposals contradict our fundamental principle—that the patient has the answer. But the motivation behind each of these statements is grounded in the feelings that the patient has been communicating; the counselor is simply using these feelings to stimulate movement and change. In reality, the counselor has no idea which decision is the best one. The key to making a proposal such as one in exercise 6.3 is remaining open to the patient's response. If the patient makes a case for the abortion, is open to a reframe, and creates a plan for coping, then she has moved toward a decision. Ultimately, the decision is hers; it is never yours. But if a patient cannot complete the process of informed consent, that also is her decision. You are not forcing a patient to go home against her will. You are empowering her to make a decision and appreciate its consequences. If there were ever a time where I felt that a patient would do whatever I suggested, I would be greatly concerned, and I would reflect this back to her. This indicates ambivalence of such depth that it likely cannot be resolved during a counseling session at the clinic. I would ask the patient to reschedule and give her homework for making a decision and planning for coping. While this may appear at first glance to be the counselor making the decision for the patient, if a patient cannot evidence a choice, then informed consent is impossible (see chapter 7 for a discussion of informed consent).

Ambivalent patients sometimes say, "If I leave today, I'll never come back." This statement is rich with material for discussion. Ask the patient to say more about what she means. Patients' reasons for not wanting to go home include concern that the embryo or fetus will be more developed as time goes on, an increase in cost, the loss of the ability to have a medication abortion, a change to a two-day procedure as gestational duration increases, or practical barriers to getting to the clinic. These are valid concerns. Ask your patient about any emotional reasons she has for not wanting to go home today. She may be avoiding certain feelings and may hope that having an abortion will make the feelings go away. She may be embarrassed or afraid to admit that she actually wants to continue the pregnancy. Or she may think that it makes her a better person to feel terrible about having an abortion. In considering all the women who have said to me, "If I leave today, I'll never come back," some did go ahead and leave without having the abortion, and some stayed and had the procedure, but in both cases, the patients found their own voices and made their own decisions. I have found that the patients whom counselors engage in a deeper level of conversation about their ambivalence tend to experience a positive transformation during their time at the clinic. Almost without exception, these patients go out of their way at the end of their stay to thank their counselor for helping them to think about themselves and their decisions in a different way.

Reality Check

Sometimes, you may need to let a patient know that the clinician cannot and will not provide an abortion (or place laminaria) for someone who is not sure of her decision. Informed consent is a legal obligation in the practice of medicine. No clinician will provide an abortion for a patient who does not consent. That can be a relief for some women. For others, it can be upsetting. A reality check also includes a consideration of how much time the patient has left for her decision before she is too far into the pregnancy to have an abortion at your clinic (or at any clinic) and how the price and method of her abortion will change as time goes on.

Owning a Decision

The decision as to how to resolve a pregnancy brings women down a road that forks at the end—one path must be chosen. For some, no path is desirable or feels like a good decision, but one must eventually emerge as the best one. This realization can be comforting. It gives permission for a patient to acknowledge that continuing the pregnancy may not be a positive option either. Her decision will be the one that has the most positives and fewest negatives associated with it. It is the decision that she is most willing to live and cope with. If she is unable or unwilling to decide, the decision will make itself—she will no longer be able to obtain a legal abortion. Not making a decision is, paradoxically, a decision to continue the pregnancy.

Case Example 6.3

Counselor: What was it like to make the decision to have an abortion?

Patient: It was hard.

Counselor: What made it hard?

Patient: I've been going back and forth about this for a few weeks. I just can't decide what to do.

Counselor: Thank you for sharing your feelings. I'm glad you were honest. Part of my role here is to help you think about what you want to do. Let's go back to when you first found out that you were pregnant. How did you find out?

Patient: Well, I went to the emergency room because I was sick. I thought that I had some sort of illness, but they did a pregnancy test and told me that I was pregnant.

Counselor: How did you feel when you found out?

Patient: Well, at first I was happy; I thought I was going to keep it. Then I told my boyfriend; he was not happy at all. He told me that he wanted me to have an abortion.

Counselor: What did you think about his reaction?

Patient: It made me think about having an abortion. It's true that we don't have a lot of stability. He lives with his parents, and I live with my sister and her husband. But I don't really believe in abortion.

Counselor: What have you thought about abortion before?

Patient: I thought that it wasn't right to kill your baby.

Counselor: When you think about abortion for yourself now, does it seem like killing a baby?

Patient: Yeah, kind of.

Counselor: Does it seem like the same thing as killing a newborn baby?

Patient: Yeah.

Counselor: You're seven weeks pregnant right now. Do you know how developed your pregnancy is?

Patient: Not really.

Counselor: Well, your pregnancy is still considered an embryo. It is smaller than half an inch.

Patient: Oh.

Counselor: What did you think it looked like?

Patient: I thought that it was like a fully formed baby.

Counselor: It's actually at a much earlier stage of development. Why don't I take a moment to explain to you how an early abortion is performed? Then I'll tell you about the safety of abortion. These two things usually help people make a decision.

* * *

Counselor: So how are you feeling now after hearing about the procedure?

Patient: I feel a lot better.

Counselor: Let me ask you a question to get an idea of how you're feeling about your decision: On a scale from one to ten, if one is being sure that continuing the pregnancy is the best decision and ten is being sure that abortion is the best decision, where are you now?

Patient: Oh, I feel like an eight or a nine.

Counselor: That sounds like you are feeling pretty sure that abortion is the best way for you.

Patient: I do. I'm not in a place in my life where I can take care of a child.

Counselor: I'm curious—what do you think is getting in the way of you being a ten?

Patient: Well, probably just my irritation with my boyfriend.

Counselor: Can you say more about it?

Patient: I'm disappointed because of how this has affected our relationship. I'm sad. [*Starts crying*] I'm realizing that he's not the person that I thought he was!

Counselor: A lot of times pregnancy really shines a light on the relationship, and it's not always what we want to see. I'm so sorry that you're going through this.

Patient: [*Sniffling*] Thank you. I think the relationship is over.

Counselor: Do you have friends to support you if you break up?

Patient: Yeah. I have my best friend and also my sister. She never liked him anyway.

Counselor: I want you to remember that any and all feelings that you have after an abortion are normal. Even if you have no feelings at all, that's okay, too. When you look back on this decision, remember what was going on in your life that made abortion the best way. Give yourself credit for that. Allow yourself to grieve the loss of your relationship. Rely on your friends and your sister. Does that sound like an okay plan?

Patient: Yeah, it sounds good.

Using the story and the scale, the counselor discovered the origin of the conflict—medical misinformation and disappointment in her partner's behavior. Another way to start off conversations about ambivalence is to use the certainty scale from the very beginning.

Case Example 6.4

Counselor: What was it like for you to make the decision to have an abortion?

Patient: It was hard.

Counselor: What made it hard?

Patient: Well, I love children. I have two now; one is three and the other is five. I just started back to work so that I can support them. Another child would upset everything that I've managed to put in place. But I don't want to do this. I'm not sure if it's the right thing. I've never really believed in it.

Counselor: I'm glad that you've shared this with me. You're in the right place to think about things. Let me ask you a question. On a scale from one to ten, if one is being sure that continuing the pregnancy is the best decision and ten is being sure that abortion is the best decision, where are you now?

Patient: I guess I'm a five.

Counselor: Okay, so you're really right in the middle?

Patient: Yeah, it feels that way.

Counselor: Sometimes people have a number for their head—what they *think* is best—and a number for their heart—the way they *feel*. If you think about where your head is—in other words, what you *think* is the best decision for you at this time—what number do you have?

Patient: I'm a ten.

Counselor: Okay, what number would you give for your heart?

Patient: With my heart, I'm a five.

Counselor: Okay, so with your heart you're at five. What is keeping you from being at ten?

Patient: I'm thinking about this baby and the kids that I already have. I don't feel right having an abortion. I've grown attached to the baby and part of me wants to have it. I feel movement. I've had kids. It feels like a *baby*.

Counselor: That must be really hard for you.

Patient: [*Starts crying*] It is hard.

Counselor: It's okay to cry here.

Patient: [*Crying*]

Counselor: [*Silence*]

Patient: [*Reaches for tissues*]

Counselor: What are you feeling right now?

Patient: I feel sad.

Counselor: Do you know what your sadness is about?

Patient: I just feel like I'm doing something wrong. The baby is innocent. What kind of person am I?

Counselor: You're expressing some very important feelings. Having an abortion in the second trimester brings up feelings like this for other women, too.

Patient: [*Dries her eyes*]

Counselor: You said that you felt like you were doing something wrong. Can you say more about that?

Patient: I feel guilty.

Counselor: Do you know where the guilt is coming from?

Patient: I feel so selfish. People say that abortion is selfish. If I cared about the baby I wouldn't do this.

Counselor: I've talked with a lot of women who felt selfish, and I've learned a lot from them. People judge when they think a person has too many children and they judge when a person has none. They call both of those things selfish. What I hear you saying is that you love children and are doing everything you can to keep the delicate balance of your family in place. You have a lot going on. You have a lot of responsibility caring for your children. They need you to be there for them.

Patient: That's true.

Counselor: You also said that you feel the baby is innocent and having the abortion makes you question yourself as a person. Can you say more about that?

Patient: The baby didn't ask to be created and now it's not asking to die. All of this is because of my mistake of getting pregnant.

Counselor: I'm really struck by the tremendous responsibility that you are placing upon yourself as the cause of others' suffering. I imagine that you did not set out to be in this situation.

Patient: No, I didn't.

Counselor: When we make mistakes we don't necessarily do so to cause suffering for ourselves or for others. Making mistakes is part of being human. When we're faced with each new life decision we can take steps to ameliorate or reduce suffering. You're at a new decision point now. You can think about which way is the best for all involved.

Patient: I feel like a lot of things point toward the abortion, but I just don't know whether I can go through with it. When I think about it, I get so upset.

Counselor: It's important that you really honor those feelings, and I'm glad you're sharing them. Let me ask you something. During this time that you were making a decision, what did you think about continuing the pregnancy?

In this example, the counselor started with the certainty scale. It would have been just as appropriate to start with the patient's story. If the counselor had started with the patient's story, she might already know a little bit about the patient's pros and cons of continuing the pregnancy. By asking what got in the way of continuing the pregnancy, the counselor begins gathering information on the six dimensions. There are many ways to gather the same information.

Patient: Well, my ex-husband did say that he would help me. He has kids with his wife, but he offered to help me if I decided not to have the abortion. My dad recently moved back to the area and said he would help too.

Counselor: What might be good about these offers of help?

Patient: Well, I could have the baby. I wouldn't have to have the abortion. But I'm not completely sure that it's the best idea.

Counselor: Tell me more about what you're thinking.

Patient: Well, there's the father of the baby. He's doing a lot of drugs and it took a lot of work to get him out of my life. I got a restraining order against him. If he knew I was pregnant, he would go crazy. If he knew I was having an abortion, he would completely flip out.

Counselor: Has all of this been part of your reasons for considering abortion?

Patient: Definitely.

Counselor: What about adoption? Have you thought about asking your ex-husband or your dad whether one of them would consider adopting the baby?

Patient: We actually talked about that, too. My ex-husband said that he and his wife would do it. I trust them, and I think I might even be able to handle it emotionally. I would do that before I would place my baby with someone not in my family. I know that I could never do that.

Counselor: Do you see any possible downside to placing the baby with your ex-husband?

Patient: Actually, no. I like his wife. He supported me in getting the restraining order. He and I are getting along a lot better now since I am getting my life together. But it's this thing with the father of this baby. He's crazy, and it's not safe to be around him. It's not that I think he'll try to get custody, but he'll try to make my life hell in the process.

Counselor: That makes me think of another way that you could think about the abortion. Besides needing to care for and sustain your own family, by having an abortion you are trying to avoid a potentially unsafe situation. That's another way that you would be thinking about the well-being of others. Have you thought about it that way?

Patient: I have. I have tried to make myself feel better by thinking about it as the safest way to go for everybody. That's probably what made me come to my appointment today. But I still feel terrible. I don't know which way is the right way to go!

After the conversation has been going on for a while, it can be helpful to reflect back her reasons for having the abortion versus continuing the pregnancy. You are there to help her hear her own reasoning so that *she* can make a decision. Remember, her story is the conversation. You don't have to come up with any material! Listen to her story, and then put forward and dwell with different possibilities.

Counselor: Here's what I'm hearing. You have several reasons for having this abortion. You have a very delicate situation here in terms of your family's financial stability, your safety, and the safety of your children. If you decide that abortion is the best decision, you and I can talk about ways to think about the abortion that can help you forgive yourself. That way, you'll be able to frame it in a way that is positive.

Patient: [*Listening*]

Counselor: It also sounds like there is a real possibility here for you to continue the pregnancy. If you want to parent the baby, you have your dad's support. If you realize adoption is best, you could approach your ex-husband and his wife because you trust that they would be good parents. The best option is the one that *you* decide is best based on all of the things that are going on in your life at this time. That's all that counts.

Patient: Okay.

Counselor: Today, you are twenty weeks pregnant. You are able to have an abortion at our clinic until twenty-four weeks. It might not be a bad idea for you to go home today and think about everything we have talked about and talk things over again with your ex-husband. I'll give you some homework to help you get more clarity on the things you and I have talked about. We'll reschedule your appointment for next week. You can come or you can cancel if you still need more time or if you have changed your mind. At any time you can call me at the clinic if you need help thinking through something. Going home today is something that women do when they're not quite sure what to do.

Patient: [*Nodding*] I think that's what I need to do.

In case example 6.4, the patient presented possibilities for both parenting and adoption. Although she had clearly thought about them before coming to the appointment, she had not fully rejected them. Sometimes coming to the clinic and talking with someone who is unbiased and nonjudgmental allows a new perspective on what is possible. As patients move out of ambivalence, they slowly build a case for one option over the others. Sometimes the patient will conclude that nothing would make it possible to continue the pregnancy or place the child for adoption. If that is really the case, then you need to (re-) explore her negative feelings about abortion, see whether she is receptive to a reframe, and come up with a plan for coping. The more ambivalent a patient is, the more time she will need to spend dwelling with different pregnancy options. If an ambivalent patient has strong negative feelings about the abortion but hasn't raised possibilities with regard to parenting or adoption, *you* can bring up the topic for conversation: "What if you continued the pregnancy?" "What have you thought about adoption?"

Considering possibilities and moving toward the most realistic and acceptable option is the desired outcome of dwelling. In case example 6.4, the patient presented both conflicts and possibilities (I feel like I'm doing something wrong; my ex-husband said that he would adopt the baby). The counselor took each possibility seriously and put it forward so that the patient could dwell there. The counselor also offered a reframe of abortion as a moral decision. Interestingly, the patient had already thought about abortion in this way, but it was not resonating with her. Reflect back your observation that nothing seems to have changed her feelings about abortion. You can even ask her to reflect on this lack of change. Reflecting back to the patient your impressions of her ambivalence can provide rich material for thought and discussion:

- We've been talking about alternatives to having the abortion, and you've rejected each of them. I've also put forward a different way to think about the abortion that gives some room for you to forgive yourself, but none of it seems to sit with you. Do you have any thoughts about that?
- I'm really appreciating how torn you must feel because I'm feeling really stumped, too. Do you have any thoughts about what is going on in this decision-making process that is making it so hard for you?
- It feels like maybe there is something about this decision that is coming into conflict with your sense of yourself as a person. Do you have any insight into that?

Case Example 6.5

In this case example, the patient makes a statement that sounds like a possibility, but when the counselor puts it on the table, the patient quickly rejects it. Notice how the counselor validates the patient's rejection.

Counselor: You mentioned to the nurse during your ultrasound that you weren't completely sure that abortion was the way you wanted to go. I'm glad you said that. That's why I'm here—to help you figure out what you think is best. What are some of the things that made you come to your appointment today?

Patient: I'm still in school and I want to finish. I'm broke and I don't have a job. I'm too young. But I don't want to have an abortion. My boyfriend's mom has offered to take care of the baby.

Counselor: I hear you saying that you aren't ready to become a parent but you also don't want to have an abortion. That puts you in a tough spot. What about that offer from your boyfriend's mom? What if she took care of the baby?

Patient: Oh, I don't want her to raise the baby!

Counselor: Why is that?

Patient: My boyfriend's mom has three other kids she can barely take care of. I'd be worried that she'd neglect my child. I'm not comfortable with the way she raises her children; my boyfriend did not have an easy childhood.

Counselor: Okay. So you're realizing some of your values about how children should be raised. That's very important to know about yourself. You mentioned that you don't want to have an abortion. Can you say more about that?

Sometimes a lot of what you are doing is keeping the patient company as she weighs pros and cons. Encourage her to consider each of the three pregnancy options and her reasons for and against each. Your curiosity and openness to learning about her experience and her decision-making process is what propels you to gather data on each of the six dimensions.

Case Example 6.6

Counselor: Is there any part of you that wished that during the ultrasound, the nurse discovered that you were too far into your pregnancy to be seen here?

Patient: Yeah.

Counselor: That's really interesting. That makes me wonder whether you might be wishing that someone or something else would make this decision for you.

Patient: That's probably true.

Counselor: What if I told you right now that you had to go home today and not have the abortion?

Patient: I think I'd feel relieved.

Counselor: That's a really important realization. Can you say more about that feeling of relief?

Patient: I just feel so torn. The part of me that wants this baby just wants to get out of here and not do it.

Counselor: That's the part of you that I think needs some attention. Hoping that you were too far is sometimes hoping that you don't have to be the one who has to decide. But you've also revealed that there's a part of you that wants the baby. What is going on in that part of you?

Patient: I've always wanted a second child, but I want one two years from now when I'll be done with school. I've been working on finishing college for a while now, and I'm worried that if I have another baby I'll never finish. That's what happened with my daughter. But I want another one. That's why I'm so torn.

Counselor: What might make it possible for you to continue this pregnancy?

Patient: My parents want me to continue the pregnancy. They offered to take care of the baby while I finished school.

Counselor: What do you think about their offer?

Patient: It's genuine. It would help a lot. But I'd be worried about how it would affect my relationship with my child. I want to be the parent from the beginning! Nothing seems like the right thing to do.

Counselor: You're doing a good job of getting all your feelings out, even if it's not bringing you immediately to clarity.

Patient: What do you think I should do?

Counselor: Women have asked me that before. I know that in the moment it seems like it would be great to have someone give you the answer, but the truth is that I don't know which way is best. Only you know, but sometimes it takes a little work and a little time to get there.

Patient: I know; I'm just so confused.

Counselor: What do you think about rescheduling your appointment for next week? You can either come to that appointment or you can cancel. But you can call me anytime this week if you need help thinking through something. How does that sound?

Patient: But I came all the way out here; maybe I should just get it over with.

Counselor: What would be good about having the abortion today?

Patient: I'd be done. It would be over with, and I wouldn't have to think about it anymore.

Counselor: What would not be good about having the abortion today?

Patient: I'd probably regret it. That's a feeling I can't shake. I'd probably regret it and wish that I could take it back.

Counselor: What's interesting about what you're saying is that on the surface having the abortion today appears to be a way to end the feeling of being torn, but on the other hand you're worried that you'd actually end up thinking about the abortion more—in the form of regret. That doesn't seem like a good context in which to make a decision.

Patient: No, not really.

Counselor: I think you are bringing up some important feelings that are worth paying attention to. For some people, coming here and talking to a counselor is a first step toward getting clarity on your decision. The next step is going home today, thinking about what we've talked about, and talking with your support system. How about we reschedule your appointment for next week?

Patient: I think that I should do that.

Counselor: I'm going to give you some homework that may help you clarify some of your thoughts and feelings. I'll also give you some readings that help women plan for coping after an abortion, in case you come back.

Patient: I'd really appreciate that.

Exercise 6.4

This is an exercise that you can do alone or with a partner in a role play. Either way, allow yourself time to think about and write down your answer in your counseling journal before reading on. The object of the exercise is for the counselor to listen to each of the patient's statements and decide how to best respond. If you are working in pairs, take turns being the counselor and the patient. The person in the role of counselor can practice saying her response out loud to the person in the role of patient. Discuss the counselor's response in terms of how it was received by the patient. If you are working alone, take a moment and write down your responses in your counseling journal before reading the answers. This is a complex exercise and requires some time to process how you will respond and why. Keep in mind that there is more than one correct response on the part of the counselor.

Marisol is a twenty-five-year-old woman six weeks and two days pregnant by ultrasound. On her health history, she reported one prior first-trimester abortion at age eighteen and one vaginal delivery two years ago. She is parenting her child as a single mother. Her response to the decision assessment was that she was not sure that she wanted to have an abortion.

Marisol: I'm really confused. I'm not sure if I want to have an abortion.

Question 6.1: Where should the counselor go next? Why?

Answer 6.1: It never hurts to start with validation. You can begin to develop rapport with Marisol by commending her on sharing her feelings and then reassuring her that she is in the right place to talk about her feelings. Next, the counselor can use the certainty scale to get a measurement of the patient's certainty. It would also be appropriate to start with her story. After hearing her story, the counselor can measure her certainty using the scale. For this exercise, let's start with the scale.

Counselor: I'm glad that you've expressed your feelings. You're in the right place to explore your decision. I'd like to start by getting an idea of how you're feeling about your decision. On a scale from one to ten, if one is being sure that continuing the pregnancy is the best decision and ten is being sure that abortion is the best decision, where are you now?

Marisol: I'm a five.

Question 6.2: Where should the counselor go next? Why?

Answer 6.2: First, the counselor should check in to see whether she and the patient are using the scale in the same way. Next find out whether there is a difference between her head and her heart.

Counselor: Okay, you're a five. So you're really unsure about which way to go?

Marisol: Yes.

Counselor: Okay, let's find out whether there is a difference between your head and your heart. If you thought about this decision with your head only, what number would you be?

Marisol: I'm a five.

Counselor: If you thought about it with your heart only, what number would you be?

Marisol: I'm a five there, too.

Question 6.3: Where should the counselor go next? Why?

Answer 6.3: Marisol is saying loud and clear that she is unsure. Leave the scale behind for now and ask her to tell her story. If she had given a ten for her head and a five for her heart, then the counselor could have asked her what was keeping her from being a ten with her heart. Because Marisol is ambivalent on both aspects of the scale, use the story method to gain an understanding of the pros and cons for each option and what's been going on in her life since finding out that she was pregnant.

Counselor: It sounds like you're really unsure. I'd like to understand how it's been for you since finding out you were pregnant. Let's go back to when you first found out that you were pregnant. How did you feel?

Marisol: I found out that I was pregnant about a week ago at the clinic. At first, I was happy and I drove home to tell my boyfriend. He's not the father of my daughter, but he's the father of this baby. He completely flipped out on me. He started yelling at me and telling me that people have been telling him that I've been cheating on him! It's not true, but he's convinced of it. He practically demanded that I have an abortion. The worst part of all of it was that he told me who had been saying this stuff about me. It was two of my friends.

Question 6.4: Where should the counselor go next? Why?

Answer 6.4: Take a moment to validate her anger. Who wouldn't be upset after this kind of betrayal? Beyond that, the counselor doesn't have enough of the story yet. What are Marisol's reasons for coming to her appointment today? What is the origin of her conflict with abortion? Ask her to continue with her story.

Counselor: I am really sorry to hear about that. That must be really hard for you. What happened next?

Marisol: Well, I confronted my friends about spreading these lies about me, but they didn't care. It was like they didn't even know me anymore. I went to see my boyfriend's mom, because we are tight. She wants me to keep it. She said she would help me take care of it. My mom said the same thing. You see, our families don't believe in abortion. Nobody knows that I had one before. It was not easy. I had to keep it a secret from everyone, and I was depressed for a long time. But here's the thing. I have a job, and I finally have my daughter in day care. I can barely afford it. If I have another baby right now, I don't know what I would do. I'd have to stop working and take care of both kids at home. But where will I get money?

Question 6.5: Where should the counselor go next? Why?

Answer 6.5: Again, empathize with her about her friends' betrayal and her tough situation. She is making a lot of important points that you'll need to follow up on. First, she is expressing some possible moral conflict with abortion, but you don't know the specifics yet; you only know that her family is against abortion. What does *she* think about abortion? Second, we are getting a sense of her reasons *against* continuing the pregnancy. Are there any reasons *for* continuing the pregnancy (she was happy when she first found out—what was that about)? Third, how serious are these offers of help in raising the baby?

Counselor: You mentioned that both your family and your boyfriend's family are against abortion. What do *you* think about abortion?

Marisol: I feel like I'm killing my baby. Believe me, I know that right now the baby is not the same size as my daughter was when I had her, and I know the stages of development. But I think about how much I love my daughter now. What if this baby is as wonderful as she is, and I'm deciding to kill it?

Question 6.6: Where should the counselor go next? Why?

Answer 6.6: Before exploring further her use of terms (killing), empathize with how hard this must be for her. She is also presenting an argument for which there is no answer; one never knows what one's child will be like. A lot of people who are against abortion argue, "What if your child was the next Einstein? How would you feel if you had an abortion?" Well, you could just as easily say, "What if your child became a tyrannical dictator and killed thousands of people?" It's a moot point. It doesn't take into account any of the particulars of a woman's situation or the myriad factors that contribute to the development of character.

Counselor: I can see why this is so hard for you. I always like to check in with people when they use the word *killing* because it means different things to different people. Can you say more about what you mean?

Marisol: I just feel like I'm ending a life and I feel sad about that.

Counselor: It's important to honor that sadness. You're also making some important statements about your beliefs and I appreciate your honesty. But the truth is that no one knows what kind of person their baby will become. It's an unfair burden to put upon yourself. You don't have a crystal ball, and neither does anyone else. What your concern says to me is how much you love your daughter and how much joy she brings to you. You want to be there for her to give her the care that she needs.

Question 6.7: Where should the counselor go next? Why?

Answer 6.7: Marisol's use of the word *killing* seems like more of a reflection of her sadness over the loss of what could be another wonderful child and less like moral conflict. Let's turn back to considering continuing the pregnancy.

Counselor: You mentioned that your mother and your boyfriend's mother offered to help you with raising the baby. What about that?

Marisol: I know that they have the best intentions, but they won't be able to keep that promise. I don't hold it against them, but they offered the same thing before my daughter was born, and that help never came. Don't get me wrong—they help out once in a while, but they have jobs too. They can't just drop everything and take care of a baby.

Question 6.8: Where should the counselor go next? Why?

Answer 6.8: Because Marisol is so stuck, stay with continuing the pregnancy a little bit longer. Even if these offers for help aren't realistic or acceptable, find out what might make it possible for her to continue this pregnancy.

> *Counselor:* Are there any other people who could help you if you continued the pregnancy?
>
> *Marisol:* There's no one else in my family who could help me. It's weird—there are a lot of people offering to help, but I know realistically they can't help in the way I would need it.

Question 6.9: Where should the counselor go next? Why?

Answer 6.9: Let's put forward adoption. If she rejects adoption, then we'll go back to abortion and see whether she can become more flexible in her beliefs.

> *Counselor:* What have you thought about adoption?
>
> *Marisol:* There's no way I could do it. If I have the baby, I'm keeping it.
>
> *Counselor:* That's a very common feeling that women have about adoption, and it's perfectly okay if adoption is not right for you. There's one thing I want to ask: Adoption has changed a lot over the years. Have you heard about open adoption?
>
> *Marisol:* No.
>
> *Counselor:* Nowadays, women can do an open adoption. That means that you get to pick the family who will adopt your child. That means that the child will always know that you are the birth mother. You and the adoptive family can arrange contact throughout the child's life in a way that is comfortable for each of you.
>
> *Marisol:* I still don't think I could do it.

Question 6.10: Where should the counselor go next? Why?

Answer 6.10: Validate her feelings about adoption, and reflect back what you have learned.

> *Counselor:* That's okay if adoption is not right for you. It seems like you are really stuck because you are saying that parenting and adoption are not possible for you right now, but you also don't want to have an abortion.

Marisol: You're right—I'm stuck. I just can't have this baby. I don't want to give it up for adoption, and I don't see any way that I can raise it myself.

Question 6.11: Where should the counselor go next? Why?

Answer 6.11: Marisol is getting some clarity around what is realistic for her. It is starting to sound like abortion may be the better option, but she has conflict. Reflect then reframe the decision to have an abortion and see whether she's receptive.

> *Counselor:* You are in a really tough situation. You have thought a lot about continuing the pregnancy, and you feel that adoption is not right for you at this time. If you were to have an abortion, I'm wondering whether you could see that your decision is based on your love for children. You are saying that you don't think this is the right time to bring a child into the world. You are just getting to a place where you are working and able to provide for your family. These are all things that women think about when they consider abortion.

> *Marisol:* I guess I hadn't thought about it that way.

Question 6.12: Where should the counselor go next? Why?

Answer 6.12: Ask her how she feels about the reframing. Then, return to the certainty scale to see whether there has been any change.

> *Counselor:* What would it be like if you thought about it that way?

> *Marisol:* It would help me feel better about having an abortion.

> *Counselor:* Let's go back to the scale. If you had to give me a number now, where would you be?

> *Marisol:* I feel like an eight or nine.

Question 6.13: Where should the counselor go next? Why?

Answer 6.13: It's not mandatory that a patient reach ten before having an abortion. Seek understanding of what's keeping her from being a ten, and plan for coping.

> *Counselor:* Can you say what's keeping you from being a ten?

> *Marisol:* I don't think that I'll ever get to a ten because of my love for my baby, but I feel sure that this is the best way for me to go for myself and for my daughter.

Question 6.14: Where should the counselor go next? Why?

Answer 6.14: Validate her feelings of love for this baby, and remind her that having an abortion does not mean that she loves this baby any less, it's just that she has to be able to take care of her daughter. If this is part of your practice, you could offer to help her pick a method of birth control that would allow her more control over her fertility so that she doesn't have to agonize over another pregnancy decision before she is ready.

> *Counselor:* Having an abortion doesn't take away your love for this baby. Having this abortion is a way for you to reduce the suffering of everyone involved, and that is compassionate and caring.
>
> *Marisol:* Thank you for putting it that way.

Question 6.15: Where should the counselor go next? Why?

Answer 6.15: Assess her expectations for coping.

> *Counselor:* How do you think you might feel afterward?
>
> *Marisol:* I know that I will feel sad, but I'll feel better by focusing on my daughter. I'll try to think about the abortion in the way that we talked about, like in the positive.

Question 6.16: Where should the counselor go next? Why?

Answer 6.16: Assess how she coped with her previous abortion.

> *Counselor:* How did you feel after your other abortion?
>
> *Marisol:* After my other abortion, I was very, very sad. I cried a lot. I felt this way for about two months.

Question 6.17: Where should the counselor go next? Why?

Answer 6.17: Assess how she coped with this sadness.

> *Counselor:* What things did you do to help cope with your sadness?
>
> *Marisol:* I pretty much came out of it by focusing on my life.

Question 6.18: Where should the counselor go next? Why?

Answer 6.18: Ask about other positive coping mechanisms that she uses and assess her support system. These are important parts of planning for coping.

Counselor: What else can you do to cope with feeling sad?

Marisol: Get out of the house and take walks; make sure I'm sleeping enough. I've noticed that I feel better when I do those things.

Counselor: Those are great ideas. Is there anyone in your life who could be someone you could talk to afterward?

Marisol: I have a friend from high school who had an abortion. I was there for her afterward. We've fallen out of touch, but I've wanted to reconnect with her. She's from a different circle of friends, so she doesn't know the girls who betrayed me. I think I'd like to talk to her.

Question 6.19: Where should the counselor go next? Why?

Answer 6.19: Remind her that all feelings are normal, including relief and having no feelings at all. Connect her with an after-abortion talk line.

Counselor: I just want you to know that feeling sad after an abortion is normal, and it doesn't mean that you made the wrong decision. What's going to be helpful this time is that you expect to feel sad, so it won't be as much of a surprise. Whatever you feel afterward, even if it is relief or nothing at all, keep in mind that there are other women out there who are feeling the same thing. Sometimes I like to give women the number to a talk line where they can call and talk about their feelings. It's a free call. Can I give you that number?

Marisol: That sounds good. Thank you.

Counselor: You're welcome. Thank you for sharing all of this with me. Are you ready to get some information about aftercare and sign the consent forms?

Marisol: Yes, I'm ready.

FINAL THOUGHTS

Several important resources are available for recommending to patients who are struggling with their decisions. The *Pregnancy Options Workbook* by Margaret R. Johnston (1998) is essential homework for patients just embarking on a decision-making journey or who have rescheduled their abortion appointment because they need more time. For patients whose ambivalence has its origins in emotional, spiritual, and moral conflict, suggest *Peace after Abortion* (Torre-Bueno 1997). Another important guide for making a decision can be found in Anna Runkle's 1998 book *In Good Conscience: A Practical, Emotional, and Spiritual Guide to Deciding Whether to Have an Abortion*. It contains exercises that patients can do to help move toward resolution. The talk lines Backline and Faith Aloud are available to women both before and after abortion, and the talk line Exhale is available to women after abortion.

Counseling ambivalent patients is a lot like being a detective following each new lead. Take the time to put forward each possibility that your patient raises, and genuinely consider it with her. As options are eliminated, the path to a decision has fewer and fewer detours. Be open to the possibility that your patient may realize that the best option for her is continuing the pregnancy. Also be sensitive to the fact that some women are truly unable to continue a pregnancy, even when they have significant conflict with abortion. If this is the case, help your patient make a plan for coping. Keep her company as she raises different possibilities and examines them, taking each one seriously. The nimble counselor follows the patient through twists and turns, keeps track of pros and cons, and validates her struggle. Remember that the patient has the answer to her dilemma and that the patient will make the decision as to which way to go—that is her responsibility, not yours. Be her interested and attentive guide and facilitator. A conversation with an ambivalent patient can take time and lots of your energy, attention, and focus, but stay by her side. It is worth it for you and your patient's growth and transformation.

Chapter Seven

Understanding Informed Consent

The central means of ensuring quality decision making in a medical context is through the legal doctrine of informed consent. Informed consent for medical decision making is considered a legal and ethical obligation consisting of duties and rights of physicians and patients, respectively. This doctrine is a product of litigation and has evolved over time (Roth, Meisel, and Lidz 1977; Grisso, Appelbaum, and Hill-Fotouhi 1997). The duties and rights of the physician and the patient constitute the *process* of informed consent. In many heath care settings, staff in addition to the physician (the physician's *designee*) are involved in this process. Notwithstanding differences in styles among clinics, two tasks must be accomplished (see box 7.1). First, the physician must provide information (so that the decision is informed), and the patient must give or refuse consent. In addition, the process of informed consent requires that information relevant to the patient's medical condition be disclosed to the patient in a manner that is easily understandable (Berg et al. 2001). Written, and sometimes additionally verbal, consent is required from the patient prior to treatment. Throughout this process, different teaching modalities (verbal, visual, models and diagrams, video, or group interaction) may be used to maximize the patient's understanding.

Box 7.1.   Duties and Rights of the Physician and the Patient

1. Physician's duty to disclose information and patient's right to obtain information
2. Physician's duty to obtain consent and patient's right to give or refuse consent

---

For a patient to give or refuse consent, certain requirements must be met: she must be competent; understand the purpose of the treatment, its alternatives and the risks and benefits of each; appreciate the consequences of each alternative; express a preference for a particular treatment; and do so voluntarily. These requirements are the *components* of informed consent (see box 7.2). Let's look more closely at the first component—*competence*.

Box 7.2. Components of Informed Consent

1. Competence
2. Understanding of the nature and purpose of the proposed treatment, its alternatives, and the risks and benefits of each
3. Appreciation of the consequences of a decision
4. Making the decision voluntarily
5. Evidencing a choice

Competence is a psychological and legal term describing a state of mind that consists of three abilities: the ability to reason, the ability to understand, and the ability to appreciate the consequences of one's decisions (Appelbaum and Grisso 1988). Notice how the definition of the components of informed consent and the components of competence overlap (see box 7.3). It can be challenging to distinguish the components of informed consent from the state of being competent to *give* consent. The truth is that there is a great deal of commonality. Competence can be thought of as a capacity that a person has, subject to change across time, wherein she can demonstrate each of these three abilities.

Box 7.3. Competence

1. The ability to reason
2. The ability to understand
3. The ability to appreciate the consequences of a decision

Beyond the abilities of competence, the literature consistently describes two other components of informed consent: that the patient is making the decision voluntarily (Scherer 1991) and that the patient can give evidence of her decision. Therefore, the process of informed consent includes the three abilities of what it means to be competent, plus two other requirements: that the decision be made voluntarily, and that the patient, in some form, be able to state her decision. Let's look at each of the components of informed consent in more detail.

COMPONENTS OF INFORMED CONSENT

Competence

Competence is sometimes referred to as the capacity for rational reasoning (Grisso et al. 1995). Rational reasoning is the ability to engage in a process of analyzing different factors and aspects of a situation in order to arrive at a decision. Rational reasoning is more concerned with a person's capacity to engage in the activity of problem solving; it does not judge the accuracy or reasonableness of the grounds that were used to arrive at a decision. Rational reasoning also does not make judgments concerning the quality of the actual decision; it is instead focused on the process employed.

Understanding

When one is capable of understanding, one can comprehend the nature and purpose of a particular medical treatment and the nature and purpose of any alternatives. Patients with the capacity for understanding know that the purpose of an abortion is to terminate a pregnancy and that after an abortion they will no longer be pregnant. They also understand that they have only one alternative—to continue the pregnancy, give birth, and parent or place the child for adoption. When states pass legislation for new informed consent policies in abortion provision, they often target this component. For example, states have enacted laws that mandate that patients be shown ultrasound images or submit to descriptions of fetal development (Gold and Nash 2007). Proponents of these laws argue that patients are not being given full information prior to their abortions and that if they could see images of the developing embryo or fetus, they might change their minds. Opponents of these laws believe that women are fully aware of the consequences of their decisions and that the true purpose of these laws is to shame women into continuing their pregnancies. What's interesting to consider is that we never hear about legislation to mandate discussions of the *risks* of childbirth or extol the *benefits* of abortion.

Understanding also requires comprehension of the risks and benefits of each alternative to the proposed treatment. This is the most concrete aspect of informed consent. It consists of a list of the risks of having an abortion (also known as complications) and the likelihood of occurrence of each. The same can be done for complications resulting from childbirth. The idea behind discussing the potential complications of each alternative and their likelihood of occurrence is that it creates an even playing field within which to weigh pros and cons of a medical decision. Because the health risks of abortion and childbirth are both quite rare, this can be a source of confidence for counselors. It's empowering to be able to reassure patients how safe abortion actually is—safer even than childbirth.

It's interesting to consider what parts of the consent form, if any, make counselors feel uncomfortable, and why. Some counselors probably minimize a discussion of risks out of a desire not to scare the patient ("Don't worry, no one ever gets a hysterectomy") or quell anxiety by falling back on anecdotal experience ("I've worked here for a year and I've never seen anyone have a cervical tear"). These anxieties on the part of staff are normal. We're unaccustomed to speaking frankly with others about the possibility of serious complications or even death. We may feel embarrassed that the service that we are providing has possible negative consequences. In our role as caregivers, we don't want to add to the patient's anxiety.

Exercise 7.1

In our role as abortion providers, we quickly come to feel secure about the safety of abortion; we can forget that it's not so obvious to our patients. Unless you've had surgery before, you also may not have thought about what information *you* would want in order to make an informed decision. Exercise 7.1 illustrates how questions about safety and risk arise spontaneously when we are confronted with a novel situation. It gives the reader an opportunity to see what arises organically in terms of concern about risk. This exercise is fun to conduct in a group format with a facilitator who can document questions and answers, but it may also be conducted by the reader alone.

The facilitator can begin by reading the following paragraph:

> For this exercise, imagine that I have built an aircraft out of 100 percent recycled material. You are invited to take a trip on this aircraft. Each of you will be transported to your family's home within seconds, where you can spend the weekend. The appeal of this new aircraft is that it eliminates the burden of travel time.

If you are the facilitator, you'll take the role of engineer and pilot. Read the questions to the group and encourage spontaneous response. After each question, I provide a discussion on how staff responded when we conducted this exercise at my place of work. Keep in mind that the order and format of the questions I have included in the exercise are based on the responses of my coworkers. Therefore, you'll need to respond to your group's questions in the order in which they arise. The important point is that you create a space for participants to express what comes to mind about risk. If you are doing this exercise alone, take a moment to write down your response to each question in your counseling journal before reading the discussion.

Question 1: What is the first question that you would like to ask about my aircraft?

Discussion: When we conducted our group exercise, Julie spoke up without hesitation and asked, "Is it safe?" This is exactly the question that I was hoping someone would ask first. I responded to the group that it was "Pretty safe."

Question 2: Let's imagine that your first question was, "Is it safe?" Here's my answer: "It's pretty safe." Are you satisfied with my response? Why or why not?

Discussion: The group wasn't satisfied, which was good. I urged them to keep interrogating me. Luz said, "How safe?" When I asked Luz why she asked, "How safe?" she stated that it was hard to feel confident or secure about a statement as vague as "Don't worry, it's safe," or "It's pretty safe."

Question 3: What would help you to understand how safe it was? Why?

Discussion: Selena spoke up, "Compared to a commercial aircraft, tell us how safe it is." This is an excellent response. Selena was asking for a context in which to understand risk. For example, most of us drive an automobile every day. We know that statistics show it is one of the riskiest behaviors that we engage in every day, but we do it anyway. It can be helpful to compare different health risks to the risk of death by an automobile accident because almost everyone can access their sense of the riskiness of riding in an automobile and how willing they are to assume that risk. The same is true for the risk of flying. I told the group that it was "safer than a flight in a commercial aircraft."

Question 4: What else would help you to understand how safe it was? Why?

Discussion: Naturally, the group wanted numbers, which impressed me. I was obliged to make up some statistics on the spot. I told them that if there were two commercial aircraft crashes per one million flights, there was only one crash per one million flights of my craft.

Question 5: How do statistics help you in making your decision?

Discussion: The group members agreed that they each knew how they felt about airline travel and if my craft was actually safer than airline travel, then they knew exactly how they felt about its safety. Being able to compare the rate of crashes between my craft and commercial aircraft gave them a sense of the reality of the risk. This was better than just saying, "It's safer than a commercial aircraft."

Question 6: Here's another piece of information. There are three possible negative outcomes to flying in my aircraft. The first is that your fingernails might turn green, but this will revert to normal a few hours after you land. The second risk is that you might get sunburn, especially if you are of a lighter complexion. The third risk is that you might go permanently blind. What would help you make more sense of these risks?

Discussion: There was a moment of silence, and then Chris spoke up. "Are there any differences between these risks? Is my risk of green nails the same as my risk of going blind?" She hit the nail on the head. Some of the risks that I listed are more permanent and dangerous than others. People want to know the likelihood of each of their risks. They would like to be able to compare likelihoods *across* risks. I made up some statistics on the spot: 5 percent of passengers suffered from green nails, 10 percent experienced sunburn, and less than one person in one hundred thousand experienced blindness.

Question 7: Given that the risk of sunburn is so high, what would you want to know about it?

Discussion: Ana asked, "Is there any way to prevent it?" I told her that I would provide sun block for each customer, thus preventing sunburn in almost all cases. Other pertinent questions from the group were whether there were differences in the severity of sunburns in terms of degree and healing time. My responses illustrated how there can be degrees of severity within the same complication.

In the end, each participant in exercise 7.1 agreed that she was in a better position to decide whether to travel on my aircraft and felt less trepidation and more empowered to make an informed decision. I reviewed with the group what had taken place during this process:

1. Possible bad outcomes (complications) can result from any decision that we make.
2. The safety of a novel situation becomes more comprehensible when we compare it to a more familiar situation.
3. We are interested in learning not only a list of potential complications, but also about the *likelihood* of each complication's occurring.
4. It reduces our anxiety when we learn ways to *prevent* complications from occurring.

Questions regarding safety and risk arise spontaneously when we are confronted with decisions that involve unknowns and novel situations. Patients may have some of the same types of questions about the safety of abortion as you did during this exercise. Think about the process of informed consent in your clinic. How well do the content, structure, and process of your clinic's

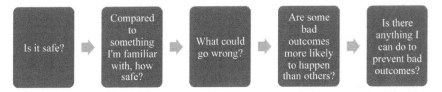

Figure 7.1. Reasoning about Risk

consent forms address the components of reasoning about risk illustrated in figure 7.1?

Appreciation of Consequences

The third component of informed consent is the ability to appreciate the consequences of one's actions. In this component, the patient imagines the impact that each alternative (abortion, adoption, and parenting) would have on her life. Appreciating the consequences of a decision could take the form of:

1. Having thought about the physical experience of having an abortion or going through childbirth.
2. Having contemplated the effect of a baby or an abortion on her relationship with her partner.
3. Having considered the bearing on her emotional well-being of having a baby, placing a baby for adoption, or having an abortion.
4. Understanding her partner's or her family's desires with regard to this pregnancy.
5. Expression of her beliefs about abortion and how those may differ from others' beliefs.
6. Recognition of her own readiness to be a parent and an acknowledgment of how a baby would change her life plans.

Appreciation of consequences can be demonstrated when a patient talks about her *reasons* for having an abortion. She may do this as a result of your asking her what it was like for her to make her decision. I'm not a big fan of asking patients *why* they have chosen abortion; it can seem patronizing and might put them on the defensive. I'm more concerned with their certainty, voluntariness, and any conflicts they might have. Patients express appreciation of consequences when they make statements such as:

- I know that I can't afford another baby right now.
- I'm not ready emotionally to be a parent right now; I'm too young.
- I'm worried that if I have an abortion, I'll regret my decision.

- My partner is physically abusive; having a child with him would tie me to him forever.
- I considered open adoption, but I realized that it's not for me.

Voluntariness

The fourth component of informed consent is the element of voluntariness. This means that the decision to have an abortion is the patient's own decision and not a result of pressure or coercion from another person. Examples of coercion are a parent forcing a daughter to have an abortion or a husband demanding that his wife have an abortion. Women and girls experiencing intimate partner violence may report that their partners are forcing them to have an abortion. Women and girls involved in human trafficking also come to the clinic under complex coercive circumstances. Be aware that the opposite can also be true— a partner or parent may be trying to force the patient to continue the pregnancy. Parental influence on a child's medical decisions often arises in the context of abortion counseling and can be one of the most complicated situations that you will face as a counselor (Scherer and Reppucci 1988). Because of the prevalence of laws requiring that one or both parents come with their daughter to the clinic and sign the consent form (or be notified by mail before the abortion), counselors in most states are likely to have faced situations where they were concerned that a teenager was being coerced into having an abortion.

A national survey asked teens under eighteen whom they had told about their abortion; 61 percent said that one or both parents knew (Henshaw and Kost 1992). So what about the other 39 percent? Why didn't they tell a parent? Here are some of the answers that they gave: 18 percent worried that a parent would make them leave home, 14 percent feared a parent would make them continue the pregnancy, and 6 percent thought they would be physically abused. The teens were also asked about discussions they had with their parents about what to do about being pregnant. While 85 percent of the mothers discussed the abortion option with their daughters, only 45 percent discussed parenting or adoption. Most concerning was the subset of the 61 percent whose parents knew about the abortion but found out through someone else besides the teen herself. Of these teens, 18 percent said their parents were forcing them to have the abortion.

This last statistic is concerning. Did they disclose this in counseling? What did the teens mean by "forcing?" There is a big difference, legally and psychologically, between parents strongly voicing an opinion in favor of abortion versus threatening their child with abuse, abandonment, or neglect if they elect to continue a pregnancy. Consider also that a teen may report that she was forced to have an abortion because she doesn't want to take ownership of her decision. Nevertheless, these data underline the importance of decision assessment and counseling with teens and their parents. Equally critical is the need for counselors to examine their own values about teen parenting. Counselors who think that teens are incapable of parenting may be less likely to assess their decisions and more likely to ignore conflict.

Evidencing a Choice

The final component of informed consent is called evidencing a choice. This simply means that the patient has provided evidence, in written form, verbal form, or both, of the decision she is making. Evidencing a choice occurs in the act of signing the consent form or in a "time out" before surgery where the patient is asked to state, in her own words, the procedure that she expects to have.

CHILDREN'S COMPETENCE TO CONSENT

Much has been written on guidelines for informed consent and the theory behind them, and a number of studies have measured competence to consent to research and treatment. The majority of those have focused on ways to assess the competence of psychiatric patients to consent to treatment and research (Grisso and Appelbaum 1995), children's competence to consent to psychotherapy (Melton, Koocher, and Saks 1983), and children's competence in hypothetical medical treatment contexts (Lewis 1981; Weithorn and Campbell 1982). One of the issues in which competence to consent has been hotly debated is in the context of minor adolescents and abortion. Whether minors are as capable as adults to meet the requirements of informed consent is a topic of much controversy in both the courts and social science research (Steinberg et al. 2009). Each state has different medical emancipation statutes that identify certain circumstances wherein minors are deemed competent to consent to their own medical care. Distinguished by their advanced age or life situation, emancipated minors can independently seek care for medical situations such as substance abuse, mental health, and reproductive health care (Crosby and English 1991). It is predominantly in the context of abortion that minors' competence has been so rigorously questioned. Lawmakers have assumed that in the case of abortion, minors are more likely to make bad decisions and suffer more severely the consequences of bad decisions than are adults. Justifications used by courts to deny minors' rights to consent for an abortion are based on several assumptions about abortion that have not been supported by research.

It is interesting to take a deeper look into why so many states have parental involvement laws. On face value, the laws seem logical. Most parents would want their daughters to tell them if they were to become pregnant and would want to be a part of helping them with that decision. Readers who are parents probably find it heartbreaking to imagine their daughter sitting in a clinic waiting room alone, not having felt that she could tell them that she needed an abortion. It is reassuring to know that most minors *do* tell a parent about their pregnancy and involve them in their decision; this is true for minors in states with and without parental involvement laws (Henshaw and Kost 1992). It is important to remember the reasons that teens feel they cannot tell a parent. Many teens are worried about repercussions of a parent finding out that they are having sex, let alone that they want an abortion. Teens who fear severe negative consequences need to be able to seek abortion care without the fear of being forced to continue the pregnancy. Laws exist to protect the most vulnerable. Abortion counselors are there to ensure that the decision is not coerced. There is no parallel context where a "parenting counselor" goes house to house, ensuring that every continued pregnancy is voluntary, uncoerced, and not a result of a lack of access to abortion care.

The stated goals of parental involvement laws are two: first, to protect vulnerable, immature minors from making unsound decisions and, second, to promote family involvement in children's medical decisions. Furthermore, these two goals are based upon three assumptions: (1) that minors are more vulnerable than adults to negative psychological outcomes after abortion and that abortion is more psychologically detrimental than carrying an unwanted pregnancy to term; (2) that minors' decision-making skills are immature and their judgment is poor; and (3) that parental involvement in an abortion decision is paramount to encouraging and maintaining family unity (Melton 1987). These assumptions have not panned out in the research on adolescent decision making and abortion. While minors may be less comfortable with their decision than adult women, they are not at risk of severe negative psychological outcomes (Major et al. 2000). In addition, research has shown that *voluntary, ongoing* communication between a parent and a daughter about sexual health has a more powerful effect on minors' willingness to consult their parents should a need for confidential services arise than state-mandated, one-time conversations (Perrucci, Schwartz, and Sigafoos 2007).

COERCION AND ADOLESCENTS

Pregnancy in adolescence magnifies family power dynamics and elucidates the struggle for autonomy and agency that occurs between a teen and her parents. The ability to assert independence in a pregnancy decision can be an important part of exercising autonomy during the teenage years. Case example 7.1 describes a teen who states she is being forced to have an abortion by her mother. The counselor has two initial tasks: to assure the teen that she cannot be forced to have an abortion and to engage in reality testing around her decision to continue the pregnancy.

Case Example 7.1

Counselor: How are you doing with your decision to have an abortion?

Teen: I don't want to have an abortion at all. I don't want to be here. My mom dragged me here today. It's her idea for me to have the abortion.

Counselor: It must have been really hard for you to come here.

Teen: Yeah, I was so pissed.

Counselor: I'm really glad that you told me and that you were honest with me. I want you to know that no one can force you to have an abortion. You have the right to continue this pregnancy, no matter what anybody else wants you to do. I'm proud of you that you had the courage to tell me that. Now let's talk a little more about how you've been feeling about being pregnant.

After validating the difficulty of the patient's situation, the first thing that the counselor communicates to the patient is that she will not be receiving an abortion if she does not want one. This single statement likely will result in a palpable decrease of tension in the room. Next, the counselor seeks to understand how the patient has been feeling about being pregnant. She takes the patient at her word and is interested in learning about the patient's feelings about pregnancy and parenthood. For some teens, just being able to say that they don't want the abortion and to be taken seriously is a huge first step toward getting clarity about what they really want. They may even be able to get clarity within the counseling session; just letting a patient know that no one can force her to have an abortion can return her sense of control. A teen may also benefit from the opportunity to talk to her mother about how she felt being "dragged to the clinic." These conversations often are best facilitated by the counselor.

The next step is reality testing about parenthood. It is imperative that the counselor discuss the possibility of continuing the pregnancy and parenting without being dismissive or patronizing. It helps to have examined your values about teen parenthood (see chapter 8). You may find yourself thinking, "But she's only fourteen!" or "This patient is way too immature to be a parent!" Recognize these are your values and opinions, not necessarily statements of fact. If you are invested in the outcome of your patient's decision, you won't be effective as an options counselor.

Reality testing means talking about matters of pure practicality:

- If she has the baby, where will she live?
- Who will cook, run errands, and do laundry?
- How will she pay for the costs of raising a child?
- Is she willing to get up every three hours during the night to feed the baby?
- Will she breastfeed?
- What does her partner think and feel? How will this shape his future?
- Are her partner's parents supportive?
- Will she be able to finish high school? Is there a teen parenting program at school?
- Does she have friends her age who have babies? How are they doing?

She will need to think through these issues and many others. This is part of "appreciation of the consequences" of a decision. No matter how far you get in this conversation, you should always send the patient home with the *Pregnancy Options Workbook* (Johnston 1998). Keep in mind that she may not even know the answers to these questions right now, but you are helping her to begin thinking about them. If you talk to her mother, you can help her come up with a plan for reality testing as well.

> *Counselor:* Let's think about what will happen today when you tell your mom that you have decided to continue the pregnancy. What do you think she is going to say?
>
> *Teen:* She's going to totally freak out. She already told me that she wasn't willing to help me. She has two jobs and is totally stressed. She's so mad right now that I am even pregnant.
>
> *Counselor:* In the past, what did your mom say she would do if you became pregnant?
>
> *Teen:* She always said that she would kick me out of the house.
>
> *Counselor:* What was it like for you when she said that?
>
> *Teen:* I was scared. But I don't think she'd actually do it; she's just mad. But I'm mad at her, too. She won't listen to me. I told her that I don't believe in abortion. She doesn't believe in abortion, either! What a hypocrite! I keep telling her, what would you do if you were in my situation? I know that she'd probably keep it. She just won't admit it.

Reality testing also means finding out why the patient is not considering abortion. In this example, the patient has begun to share some of her beliefs, but the counselor needs to better understand where her beliefs are coming from. That will provide insight into how much of her desire to continue the pregnancy is based on a desire to have a baby versus fear of the abortion or a desire to contradict her mother. Take some time to see whether there is any flexibility in her beliefs—are there circumstances where she feels that abortion is okay? Here are some examples of questions from chapter 5 for seeking understanding of beliefs and looking for flexibility.

- What are your beliefs about abortion? Where did they come from? How long have you had those beliefs?
- Can you think of any circumstances in which you think abortion is okay?
- Can you think of any aspects of your life situation that would make abortion okay?
- What have you thought about adoption?

Counselor: I can imagine that you are probably scared and worried. We'll talk about ways to tell her. If you give me permission, I can talk to her, too. But for now, let's think of where else you could live if you were kicked out. Who else in your family knows that you are pregnant?

The counselor needs to give the patient things to think through in terms of the reality of her situation. That way, the patient can go home and actually try to answer these questions and see whether having a baby is realistic and acceptable. Unless she is taken seriously and gets the opportunity to process these things, she will never be able to fully own her decision.

Counselor: I have an idea. What would you think if I talked to your mom before you leave the clinic? I would tell her that you don't want to have an abortion today. I would talk to her about ways that you and she can talk about your decision. I'll only talk to her about things that you give me permission to talk about. What do you think?

Teen: That would be great. Just don't tell her that I called her a hypocrite.

Counselor: Okay, I won't tell her that. I expect that she is going to be quite upset; she'll probably even be mad. I want to try to help her with her own feelings about what is going on. That part won't even be about you; it will be more about her. How does that sound?"

Teen: That sounds good.

Counselor: When I'm done, do you want me to bring your mom back here so you can say a few words to each other with me here?

Teen: Yes, please.

When patients state that they don't want to have an abortion, it is tempting to cancel their appointment and quickly move on to the next patient. We may want to avoid talking to a parent because we anticipate anger—remember that your patient is equally as uncomfortable and scared, if not more. I almost always receive permission from the teen to talk to her parent or other adult family member who accompanied her. Most are terrified to break the news themselves. I find it best to talk to the parent alone first. This creates a space to use level 1 skills to normalize and validate anger, frustration, and despair. Acknowledge the difficulty of the parent's struggle. Provide a new approach to talking about the teen's pregnancy decision in a way that will allow for both reality testing and respectful, honest communication. It is imperative to communicate to parents that the decision as to how to resolve a pregnancy is a critical moment in adolescent development and must be made in a context free of coercion. When talking with parents, I advise them on three things:

1. Create a space where your daughter can express her feelings and desires about this pregnancy.
2. Share your own values and life experiences with your daughter.
3. Engage in reality testing.

Always lead with empathy and compassion for the enormity of a parent's conundrum. Parents have valid reasons to be upset; learn about the reality of the family's situation. Given that your clinic will not provide an abortion in the context of coercion, parents need new ideas for communication with their children. This is the only path on which their teenager can access her true desires around this pregnancy decision.

Case Example 7.2

Counselor: Hello, Mrs. Johnson. Can I talk to you privately? Your daughter has given me permission to talk to you about some things that we discussed in counseling. She has stated that she does not want to have an abortion; she wants to continue the pregnancy.

Parent: What? What the hell is she talking about? She knows she can't raise a baby! I told her that there was no way that she was going to have a baby and dump it on me. I work two jobs. My ex-husband left me with three kids. I can barely support myself. I can barely pay my bills. I am so stressed out and now she is trying to make me completely crazy with all this talk about having a baby! This is ridiculous. She has to have that abortion today. I'm going to go in there and make her.

Counselor: Mrs. Johnson, I am truly sorry. I can see that you are in a tough situation and that this is not what you want to hear at all. But give me a minute and I'll try to explain some things that might help you in this situation. But I need to emphasize that we cannot give someone an abortion when they say they don't want one.

Parent: I don't care what she wants; she has no idea how to raise a child! I can't take on a baby!

Counselor: I hear what you are saying. What I am going to try to do is help you find a way to talk with her so that *she* can figure the best decision for herself. We all know the importance of rebellion. Sometimes teens say that they want something just because they know it's the exact opposite of what their mom wants. You and I are going to come up with ways for you to talk to her so that she isn't saying that she wants to have a baby just to make you mad. When you found out she was pregnant, what did you say to her?

Parent: I told her that this household cannot support a new baby right now. She said that she agreed that the abortion was the best thing.

Counselor: A lot of parents have the same experience—their child agrees that abortion is the best decision at home, but then she changes her mind at the clinic. What we have to do is create a space for her to share what else is going on with her. Coming all the way to the appointment and then refusing to have an abortion is a big deal. I'm not exactly sure where that's coming from, but I have some ideas about how to get at it. Sometimes what daughters need is for their moms to listen to them, hear what they are saying, and take them seriously. Pregnancy and parenting are serious things, as you know. Being pregnant and deciding what to do about it is a decision where a person gets to think about serious, adult, mature issues. Some daughters, when they sense how strongly their moms want them to have an abortion, react in the opposite way in order to assert that they are serious, adult, mature people, too. Teens want to be taken seriously, and this is a place where they can create a pretty serious situation. They may not even clearly understand what they really want to do because they are so busy asserting their independence from their parents.

Parent: [*Nods*]

Counselor: I'd like to share with you three things that parents sometimes find useful in these situations. The first is that you need to create a space where your daughter can express her feelings about this pregnancy. Treat continuing the pregnancy as a real possibility, and take her seriously. Only then can she let go of the need to have a baby just to make you mad! You'll have to let go of negative feelings, if only for this conversation. The second thing I would advise you to do is talk with your daughter about *your* beliefs about teen parenting, abortion, and adoption. One thing that sometimes plays a big part in a daughter's decision to continue a pregnancy is her perception of her mother's beliefs about abortion. Have you two ever talked about your views about abortion?

Parent: No.

Counselor: I'd like to ask you a personal question. Have you ever had an abortion?

Parent: Yes, a long time ago, but I never told her. But I had my daughter when I was fourteen. Just like her.

Counselor: Thank you for sharing that with me. And yes, I think the fact that you had her when you were fourteen is probably something that is influencing her decision. How did you feel about your abortion?

Parent: I thought it was the best thing for me at the time. I still do.

Counselor: The abortion is definitely your personal business, and you have the right to decide whether you want to tell her. However, I am wondering whether talking about that experience could influence her ability to get clarity on what she wants. If she knew that you had an abortion, how you felt about it, and how it changed your life, she might come to a different understanding about abortion. Would you consider telling her?

Parent: I would consider it.

Counselor: The other important thing is how you were fourteen years old when you had her. The truth of the matter is that you know exactly what it is like to be a parent at her age. You also know that you survived and that you love your daughter. Your daughter can only benefit from a truthful discussion of what that was like for you and the circumstances surrounding your decision. At the same time, you need to assure her that when a woman considers abortion for any of her pregnancies, it doesn't mean the pregnancy doesn't have any value or meaning. It doesn't take away from the love that you have for her or your love for the baby that you didn't have. She could be thinking that if she has an abortion now, it is like saying that *she* doesn't have any value because her baby is supposed to be born just like she was born. But you have to try to show her, as you well know, that the one doesn't have to do with the other. Even though each pregnancy is unique, each pregnancy is not the same as the child once it is born and grown. If your abortion resulted in a positive change in the family, or your ability to care for your daughter, or your ability to change your life for the better, it is important to share that with her. You'll need to show her how having an abortion is a decision made out of love and compassion.

Parent: I believe that. Thank you for saying it that way.

Counselor: You're welcome. The third thing that you need to do is help her do some reality testing. You need to communicate with her about what it takes to raise a child and to what extent you will be able to help her. Let her know about all the things you are *not* able to help her with. Sit down at the kitchen table and plan this thing out. Make a list with her of all the different appointments she will need to make; give her a bus schedule and a map. Get out a piece of paper and talk about how much different things cost, and compare that to how much money is in her piggy bank. Make a list of all the things that she likes that she'll no longer be able to afford. If you have a close relative with a new baby, let her spend some time at the house. Wake her up in the middle of the night to practice getting up to feed the baby. You must do this as if there is no other option besides her continuing the pregnancy. You must do your best to do it without being angry or upset. Be kind, but be neutral. Mrs. Johnson, what do you think about all these things I have been saying?"

Parent: I'm overwhelmed, and I'm still pissed off as hell. I can't do this!

Counselor: Anyone in your situation would feel completely overwhelmed. And furious! But since you can't force her to have an abortion, you have to take a different stance. You can tell her that you are angry, but you also have to give her a chance to say how she feels. You have to let her see that you will join her in thinking about having this baby so that she can really decide whether that is what she wants to do.

Parent: What do I say to her?

Counselor: First, you need to do something for yourself. Acknowledge that you are extremely angry and that your anger is understandable and normal. Then take a deep breath and let it go for now.

Parent: [*Sighs*]

Counselor: Say to her, "I hear that you don't want to have an abortion. Well, okay. Let's go home and talk about how you are feeling and what you want to do." Let her express her feelings about this pregnancy. Next, talk about your beliefs about teenage parenting and abortion. Share your personal experiences with each. Then tell her how much she means to you and how the abortion that you had wasn't because you didn't care about the pregnancy, but was instead about how much you cared about her. Ask her to talk about her own beliefs too. Remind her that sometimes people who don't believe in abortion realize that it can be the right decision for them in certain circumstances. Mrs. Johnson, did the two of you used to be close when she was little? Have you grown apart now that she is a teenager?

Parent: Yes.

Counselor: That can happen when moms and daughters don't have enough time to share their feelings. It also happens when daughters are trying to grow up and become adults. That means sometimes not sharing as much with mom, or talking more to friends than to mom. Talk with your daughter about how much you miss talking to her and how much you love her. Those things will go a long way toward allowing her to really think about what she wants to do about this baby.

Parent: Okay, I think I can do that.

Counselor: Let's go back across the hall and get your daughter. Then you can head home and start practicing talking with each other, listening, and making decisions together.

The relationship between the abortions that a woman has and the babies that a woman has is part of the story of her life. If a teenager's mother was a teen parent, she may be pulled to justify her own existence by "keeping her baby." Counselor and parent can help the patient see that making the decision to have an abortion doesn't take away from the meaning of and love for the baby that she won't have. Having an abortion can mean the opportunity for her future children to have the best possible life. Equally true is that a teenager may decide to continue the pregnancy, and that is her right. Many women have children during their teenage years. They have wonderful families and a full life. Just because someone is young doesn't mean that she can't be a good parent. To be an effective counselor, you must not come with an agenda for your teenage patient. The decision is hers and hers alone. What you are providing is the guidance and tools for her to make the best decision for herself, and for her loved ones to provide her with a space in which to make that decision.

THE CONSENT FORM

Informed consent is a process that represents the totality of all the components of counseling that we discussed in chapter 1. While it culminates in the explanation and signing of the consent form, the work of informed consent begins much earlier. It is tempting to let the patient read the consent form on her own. Although this may provide much-needed time for charting, you lose the opportunity to ensure good comprehension. Reading the consent form together preserves the process of informed consent for a patient with poor reading skills or low literacy. Reading aloud to a patient who is following along visually also uses two learning modalities, thus increasing the chances of good understanding. Reading and explaining the consent form also provides an opportunity to incorporate and connect aftercare instructions as a means to prevent or mitigate complications (see figure 7.2). Referring back to aftercare instructions shows patients that the signs and symptoms that we ask them to look out for actually have a purpose—to diagnose complications early. "Things to look out for" takes on a clearer, more intentional meaning. When reading about the risk of infection, the counselor can refer back to the section in the aftercare instructions that lists the signs and symptoms of infection. The counselor can also point to the segment that explains the antibiotic that she will take at home, if applicable. Infusing the consent form with aftercare instructions is not only another opportunity to reinforce aftercare but also a way of making both documents more comprehensible. Patients learn not only the difference between severe pain and normal cramping but also see why it is important to look out for this symptom.

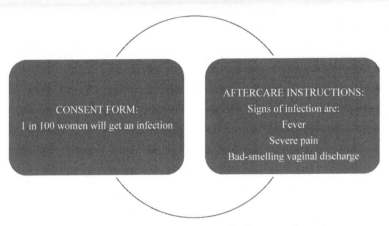

Figure 7.2. Connecting the Consent Form and Aftercare Instructions

Let's look at an excerpt from a consent form for first-trimester abortion. Consent forms often begin with an attestation of voluntary consent on the part of the patient:

> I am pregnant and do not want to be pregnant. I choose to have an abortion to end my pregnancy. My decision is voluntary. I know that I could continue the pregnancy, but I choose not to.

These basic yet profound statements allow the patient to confirm that she understands the nature and purpose of an abortion, its alternative (continuing the pregnancy), and that her decision is voluntary. This sentence addresses several components of informed consent, specifically voluntariness, evidencing and choice, and understanding the alternative to abortion.

Let's look at a second excerpt. This puts the risks of abortion in context:

> The risks of abortion are less than those of childbirth but even with careful medical care, there are possible problems.

A list of possible complications can follow this statement. When we talk about complications and their likelihoods, it is important to group those that have similar likelihood and list them from the most common to the least common. Point out to the patient that as you move down the list, they become more serious but also less common. All medical terms such as *cervical tear, perforation, hemorrhage*, and *hysterectomy* should be defined on the form (e.g., "hysterectomy, an operation to remove the uterus"), but counselors can add additional description or comments about how these are prevented or treated. The risk of death, being the least likely to occur, is listed last. There may be some initial trepidation in reading this out loud, but it will probably be short-lived. Once counselors understand why complications occur and what providers do to prevent and treat them, they, too, feel empowered. Most importantly, major complications, including risk of death, are more common in childbirth. This is a source of tremendous relief for counselors and is liberating in the sense that staff no longer have to feel apologetic or embarrassed about the possible complications of abortion.

FINAL THOUGHTS

Informed consent is an important ethical and legal component of medical decision making. Counselors play an essential role in ensuring that patients are making informed decisions. Informed consent empowers the patient by showing her that it is possible to possess the necessary knowledge to make an informed decision. The conversation between the counselor and patient is meant to be a shared learning process. As the counselor fulfills her obligation to provide information in a manner that the patient can understand, the patient feels more comfortable asking for any additional information she needs in order to provide consent. The nervousness that many staff may feel at first when talking about risks and likelihoods soon gives way to a sense of pride and empowerment as patients remark, "It's all really clear to me. Thank you for taking the time to explain everything." I find that the more complete, succinct, and clear my process, the more likely patients are to be interested, active participants. This too helps relieve their anxiety.

Chapter Eight

Decision Counseling for Positive Pregnancy Test Results

Pregnancy test counseling is the final scenario in which we'll apply our approach and framework. Like ambivalence counseling, it is imperative that the counselor follow the fundamental principle: *the patient has the answer*. It is also imperative that the counselor have no investment in or desire for the patient to choose a particular pregnancy option. In this chapter I present case examples in which the reader will learn how to nonjudgmentally guide patients through the different alternatives. In the case examples, we will analyze how the words we use communicate different things to our patients, whether intentionally or not. Therefore, we'll begin by examining our values about different pregnancy decisions in order to self-reflect on what makes us uncomfortable. This is a first step toward maintaining our approach of listening to the patient, not assuming that we share the same understanding of feelings and concepts, and reflecting on how our values affect the work that we do.

VALUES CLARIFICATION

Values clarification is an important exercise for increasing compassion and reducing burnout in direct-care settings. When our work involves facilitating behavioral change and emotional transformation, we want to be sure that we understand and clarify our own values so that our work with others is primarily about *others* and not motivated by a need to affirm our own beliefs or justify the choices that *we* have made.

Each of us holds values and beliefs that guide our behavior. Sometimes our beliefs and our behaviors are aligned, and sometimes they are not (see chapter 5 for a discussion of cognitive dissonance). Our beliefs and values affect the work that we conduct with others. They influence the words that we use, our tone of voice, and our body posture. Patients pick up on these sometimes overt, sometimes subtle communications; they can reveal compassion or negative judgment. Negative judgment diminishes rapport and decreases our effectiveness as counselors. Everyone passes judgment; the key is noticing when and how these judgments arise. Health-care providers of all kinds can usually describe a patient or a circumstance that evokes negative judgment or leaves them feeling frustrated, irritated, or angry. We can all recall situations and people who have tested our limits. These particular situations and people can move us toward burnout if we do not take the time to examine our reactions and give ourselves the space to process our feelings. The skill of holding judgment at bay comes from clarifying and deepening an understanding of values and their origins. It involves recognizing the difference between what is personally meaningful versus what is meaningful for others and respecting others' ability to make decisions in accordance with their life circumstances.

Values clarification augments self-reflection, which helps an individual to grow and develop interpersonally. By coming to terms with personal values and their impact on relationships with others, you can increase the clarity and deliberateness with which you interact with others. Values clarification—like psychotherapy and other practices that aim to develop insight through informed self-reflection—is part of the path toward wisdom (Baltes and Staudinger 2000). This means "owning your own stuff" and noticing how it tangibly influences your interactions with others. A key component of the work of the abortion counselor is an examination of personal values and beliefs about abortion, adoption, and parenting. We must discover the points where we begin to feel uncomfortable or judgmental. We must identify the places where we tune out or lose compassion. These places are different for every person. This work is an essential prerequisite for learning how to conduct effective positive pregnancy test counseling and decision counseling. Discovering personal values and bringing to light the beliefs that sustain them is not meant to create feelings of shame. Instead, the work of honest and transparent self-reflection is transformative. The more we know about ourselves—our strengths and our challenges—the more we are fully present in our relationships with others. Authentic self-reflection can also bring humility, bringing us closer to others. In the words of Brian Hatch from Berkeley Free Clinic, "You have to know what it *is* in order to leave it at the door."

A great place to start exploring values around pregnancy decisions is examining how you feel about women who have multiple pregnancies. For most people there is a number—albeit different for each person—after which one feels that a woman has had "too many" abortions or "too many" children. Granted there are some people for whom no number of abortions or children brings discomfort. Where each person draws the line for the realm of *too many* is personal. Thus the origin of the discomfort is personal; its meaning belongs to the realm of personal values.

Exercise 8.1

The work of values clarification brings the thoughts and feelings that surround different pregnancy scenarios into conscious awareness. We may feel ashamed of having certain thoughts or feelings, or we may feel self-righteous. Suspend judgment during this exercise; the first step is letting thoughts and feelings out without self-censoring. Write your answers to the following questions in your counseling journal.

1. In your opinion, how many is "too many" abortions for a woman to have?
2. Write down at least one thought and one feeling that come to mind when you think of a woman who has had that many abortions.
3. In your opinion, how many is "too many" children for a woman to have?
4. Write down at least one thought and one feeling that come to mind when you think of a woman who has that many children.

It is our responsibility as counselors to recognize and acknowledge our thoughts and feelings about pregnancy decisions and that they are not necessarily the same as those of our patients. It is often the case, however, that women feel significant negative self-directed emotions about the number of pregnancies they have had. If we agree that part of a counselor's role is to help the patient explore negative self-directed emotions, then it becomes necessary that counselors examine their negative judgments about multiple pregnancies beforehand. Let's look at some examples of thoughts that come to mind when counselors consider patients who have multiple abortions:

- How irresponsible!
- Hasn't she ever heard of birth control?
- That's a failure of the health-care system.
- I'll bet she has a lot of sex.
- That's too much disregard for human life.

Invariably, there are *feelings* that exist alongside these thoughts. Some examples are anger, frustration, disgust, and pity. Once you have isolated a few thoughts and the corresponding feelings that come up, you have begun the work to clarify your values. The second part of exercise 8.1 asks you to think about the correlative example of women who have multiple children. When you learn that someone has six children, does that mean something different to you than when you learn that she has two? Does it make a difference to you whether she is middle class or poor? Write your thoughts in your counseling journal. People's values surrounding multiple abortions and multiple births are not always the same. Some people harshly judge large numbers of children but don't care about the number of abortions, or vice versa. Other people have the same opinion of a woman who has had six children as they do of a woman who has had six abortions.

Exercise 8.2

Imagine that a patient at your clinic has received a positive pregnancy test result. As you give her the result, she becomes extremely happy. In your counseling journal, write the thoughts and feelings that arise as you imagine giving results in the following three scenarios:

1. Imagine that this patient is sixteen years old. What thoughts and feelings come to mind?
2. Imagine that this patient is thirty years old, employed, married, and has a two-year-old child. What thoughts and feelings come to mind?
3. Imagine that this patient is unmarried, receives government assistance, and has three other children at home. What thoughts and feelings come to mind?

Our values often change as the context of a woman's life changes. A counselor might react to giving results in the first context by thinking, "Having your first child at age sixteen is completely irresponsible!" What might this counselor be *feeling*? Let's imagine that one feeling is anger. What is the anger about? What pictures, images, or impressions come with the anger? She might find herself saying, "I'm angry because I think she is being irresponsible. She is a child herself. How can she care for a baby?" These statements are indications of the *counselor's* opinions and values. Given that the counselor and the patient are strangers, the counselor's response begs the question, "How does this *patient's* decision affect the *counselor's* life?" What the counselor's reaction does *not* take into account is the possibility that her teenage patient could be a good parent, that it could help her turn her life around for the better, or that during this part of her life she has optimal health and the greatest family support for child rearing.

Exercise 8.3

Let's go a little deeper. How would you respond to these questions? Write your thoughts in your counseling journal:

- So what if someone behaves irresponsibly?
- So what if a child is raised in poverty if she is wanted and loved?
- So what if a sixteen-year-old girl, who wants to have a baby, becomes pregnant?

Let's look at what you wrote in your journal. You might have said that what's wrong with being irresponsible is that it means a person is not acting like an adult, is not planning for the future, and is expecting others to take care of her problems. You might have said that raising children in poverty means that they'll never have certain opportunities or will lack certain resources. You might have said that parenthood at age sixteen robs a girl of her adolescence. Those value statements reveal a lot about your own opinions, what you want for your own life, and what you want for your own children. They also reveal a lot about your past and your future and what things are possible and available to you. But that's *your* reality. Your reality may be very different from the reality of your patient. Let's take another look at what you wrote in your journal about the "so what" statements. Can you uncover a value statement inherent in how you responded to each question? Take a moment to examine your responses before reading on. Here are some examples of values statements that represent very different values:

1. So what if someone behaves irresponsibly?
   a. People who behave irresponsibly often incur consequences that become a burden on the rest of society.
   b. Making mistakes, taking risks, and "behaving irresponsibly" is part of being human, an opportunity for learning, and a step on the path toward adulthood.
2. So what if a child is raised in poverty if she is wanted and loved?
   a. Children should be brought into this world only when parents have adequate resources to care for them.
   b. People who are poor have the same procreative rights as everyone else. The government should ensure that people who want to bear children can do so despite their socioeconomic status.
3. So what if a sixteen-year-old girl, who wants to have a baby, becomes a parent?
   a. Having a child at age sixteen robs a girl of her adolescence and her future.
   b. There is nothing intrinsically wrong about parenting during the teenage years. In fact, for some it is an ideal time in terms of health and family support. Framing teenage pregnancy as a public health problem

reflects the values of the privileged class and ignores the real problem of poverty.

Exercise 8.4

Our values originate in our experiences with our families, friends, communities, and cultures. Let's take yet another look at what you wrote in your journal about the "so what" statements. Examine your responses through the following lenses. Write your thoughts in your counseling journal.

• Think about some times that you've made mistakes, taken risks, or "behaved irresponsibly." How do you think about those times now?
• What is your experience living in poverty? How does this shape your views about raising a child in poverty? What if the patient in this scenario were never to become middle class? Should she forgo parenthood even though it's something she's always wanted?
• What is the ideal age to become sexually active? How does your personal experience inform that? How does the positive or negative quality of your experience influence what you would encourage or discourage in others?

What is normal or ideal for you is not necessarily acceptable or realistic for your patient. If you are unable to recognize this, it will inhibit your ability to establish genuine rapport or to counsel from a place of neutrality. When we work in family planning or abortion care, it is easy to become complacent in the examination of our values. This is because it is tempting to assume that openness to abortion predicts flexibility and tolerance in other areas. But we may be intolerant of women who have large numbers of children, children at a young age, or children when unmarried. Consult the work of Arline T. Geronimus (2003) on poverty, structural racism, and health and her critical analysis of the age at which women initiate childbearing. Her research and writing pinpoint how society's values about teenage childbearing presuppose economic privilege. Also refer to Kristin Luker's seminal work *Dubious Conceptions: The Politics of Teenage Pregnancy* (1995) and its critique of the framing of teenage pregnancy as a public health problem.

Some readers may contend that the origin of their values around multiple pregnancies that result in multiple births stems from concerns about overpopulation, climate change, and the dwindling supply of natural resources and that these issues affect the well-being of all of the earth's inhabitants. While these may be valid concerns, the counseling session of an individual patient making an individual life decision is not the appropriate time or place to apply them. When we find ourselves continually frustrated by the behavior of individuals and its consequences for the larger world community, it may be time to turn our focus upstream and dedicate ourselves to investigating social problems on the macro level. Many people divide their careers between providing direct care on the front lines and working upstream with a public health focus. This can be a rewarding path to take in one's professional life.

Each time you have the opportunity, ponder how your values have bearing on your work as a counselor. Strive to create a space where you can think about these pregnancy scenarios on a deeper level. Take the time to consider the meaning of your reactions and their origins. Our judgments about others' behaviors and decisions can affect our work; we may have a harder time establishing rapport with patients who push our buttons. The first step is to identify the situations that make you uncomfortable. Think freely about the things that bother you; try to think about *why* they bother you. Identify the feelings behind your explanations. Articulate the values that represent those feelings. Finally, seek to discover the origin of your values in your social or cultural upbringing. The point of values clarification is bringing the values—and their corresponding thoughts and feelings—into the light. It involves uncovering origins of sometimes deeply held beliefs. To work fully in the service of others and to experience growth and change demands that you learn about your values. It is part of the ongoing process of self-reflective living; as long as we are in relationship to others, this work is never done.

DECISION COUNSELING FOR
POSITIVE PREGNANCY TEST RESULTS

Unlike patients who present at the abortion clinic, patients who present for pregnancy testing may have no idea how they plan to resolve the pregnancy. In fact, they may have no idea whether they are pregnant! Patients in these situations often need accurate information about the three pregnancy options before they can even begin to appreciate the consequences of each. They may not know how an abortion is performed or to what gestational duration abortion is legal and accessible in their state. They may not know about open or kin adoption. Your patient may be desperate for accurate, unbiased information on these topics. You'll be the first point of contact—it is imperative that you present the options honestly and equally. Let's take a moment to review the three components of our approach in the context of counseling for positive pregnancy test results:

1. Listen.
2. Do not assume!
3. Self-reflect.

Be an active, engaged listener. This communicates interest and respect. Be curious about and genuinely concerned with the patient's well-being. If you are bored, afraid, distant, stiff, or judgmental when talking to a patient on the telephone or in person, she will instantly pick up on that and give it right back to you! You reap what you sow: the seeds that you plant in your approach to your patient determine what will grow between you. If you give respect and compassion, usually you will get it back. If you are interested in learning more about the patient, she will be more willing to share.

Don't assume that you and the patient share the same understanding of feelings and beliefs. In particular, don't assume that you and the patient share the same understanding of medical terms. When you report test results, provide an explanation of what they mean. Don't assume how she'll feel about positive results or that you fully understand her reaction to her results—ask her to say more about it. Find and follow her feelings; seek to understand them better. Look at the expression on her face. Be aware of her body posture. Listen to the words that she uses. What is she communicating? Don't assume that you understand what she means when she expresses a feeling. Ask her to say more about it. Don't assume that you understand the origin of her feelings. Ask her to say where a feeling is coming from. Finally, to be an effective pregnancy test counselor, you must spend time engaging in values clarification. Complete exercises 8.1–8.4.

Before Disclosing Results

Sometimes patients come with expectations and hopes for a particular result. They may also know exactly what they want to do if the results are positive. The best way to prepare for disclosure of results is to get a sense of the patient's desires *before* disclosure (see box 8.1). If you have the opportunity to meet the patient before conducting her test, seek out a private space to ask a few questions about what she is expecting.

Box 8.1.   Questions to Ask before Giving Test Results

- What do you *think* the results will be?
- What are you *hoping* the results will be?

Case Example 8.1

Counselor: I'm Alissa, and I'm going to do your pregnancy test. I'll also be the person who brings you the results. Tell me, do you have any idea what the results might be?

Patient: Yeah, I'm worried that it will be positive.

Counselor: Did you take any other pregnancy tests before today?

Patient: Yeah. I did a home pregnancy test two days ago.

Counselor: What were the results?

Patient: It was positive.

Counselor: Okay, that gives us an idea of what to be prepared for today. No matter what the result is today, I'm here to talk with you about your options and help you make a plan.

When you come back into the room to give this patient her positive result, you can move directly to ascertaining her feelings and thoughts about it. You're more prepared because you know a little bit about what she *expects* and what she *wants*. In this example, the counselor could have continued this conversation by seeking understanding of the patient's worry and her feelings about her home pregnancy test results, but it is also appropriate to conduct the test and then return afterward to initiate a deeper conversation. Sometimes patients will have no idea what the result will be. Instead, ask them what they are *hoping* the results will be.

Case Example 8.2

Counselor: I'm Alissa, and I'm going to do your pregnancy test. I'll also be the person who brings you the results. Tell me, do you have any idea what the results might be?

Patient: I have no idea.

Counselor: Have you had unprotected sex with a man since your last period?

Patient: Yeah.

Counselor: Have you had any symptoms that lead you to think you might be pregnant?

Patient: No.

Counselor: How about your periods? Are they regular?

Patient: Yes.

Counselor: Have you missed any periods?

Patient: Yeah. I missed my period this month.

Counselor: Okay, so that was a change in your body for you. You were smart to come to the clinic today to find out whether you are pregnant. Tell me, what are you hoping the results will be?

Patient: I'm praying that it will be negative.

Counselor: What would be bad about it being positive?

Patient: There is no way that I can have a baby right now.

Counselor: Okay. No matter what the result, I will give you information and help you make a plan. We'll hope for a negative result, but if it's positive we'll work through a plan together.

Patient: Thanks for being so understanding.

One of the most common complaints that I hear from patients at the abortion clinic are stories about *how* staff at the facility where they obtained their pregnancy test disclosed their pregnancy test results. These stories have a common theme—the way that staff reacted to positive results. Staff will exclaim, "Congratulations!" and show ultrasound images without asking patients whether they want to see them. When patients state that they do not want to continue the pregnancy, they are met with silence, disdain, and judgment. Some patients keep their plans for abortion to themselves for fear of being stigmatized. Thus, they receive no information or referrals to the nearest abortion provider.

Disclosing Results

Exercise 8.5

The words and tone of voice that you use to disclose pregnancy test results have a direct effect on your patient's experience. Consider how the counselor in this exercise reports pregnancy test results to the patient:

> *Counselor:* Your pregnancy test result came back positive. So, do you want to keep the baby or not?

Let's examine the counselor's statements through the lens of our approach. Take out your counseling journal and document your answers to each question.

1. What assumptions do the counselor's statements make?
2. In what ways do the counselor's statements create a space for the patient to disclose what she is thinking and feeling? In what ways do they not create this kind of space?
3. What could this counselor's statements be revealing about her own biases toward particular pregnancy options? Which words communicate that bias? Why?

The counselor's statements in exercise 8.5 are a common way of disclosing results; unfortunately, they do not create an open, unbiased space in which patients can reveal what they are thinking and feeling. Instead, they close down avenues of thought and discussion. An important point of concern is that the first statement assumes that the counselor and patient share the same understanding of medical terminology and the meaning of a *positive* pregnancy test. Here's an alternative way to disclose results that avoids confusion:

> *Counselor:* I have the results of your pregnancy test. The test came back positive; that means you are pregnant.

After disclosure of results, allow a moment for the information to sink in. Be silent and watch your patient's face for emergent feelings. Resist the temptation to immediately fill the space between the two of you with words, factual information, and closed-ended questions. In the silence, allow your curiosity to grow about how she will respond—remember that you are there as her support and her guide. Disclosing pregnancy test results clearly and nonjudgmentally can be accomplished in two or three sentences, but the content of these sentences—as well as the tone of voice and bodily comportment with which they are delivered—communicates a lot to the patient. If the patient begins to communicate feelings through tears, facial expressions, or changes in her posture, validate and normalize, and then seek understanding of her experience. There are many ways to ask open-ended questions that create a space for feelings. Even if you don't see any evidence of feelings, it is still a good idea to ask the question.

- What are you feeling right now?
- What's coming up for you?
- What are you thinking about right now?
- What's going through your mind?
- What's going on inside?

After you hear or see a feeling, it's still best not to assume that you understand the personal meaning of that feeling. Move to level 2 and ask your patient to say more about it. Remember to return to level 1 to validate and normalize any new feelings that you see or hear.

> *Patient:* [*Starts to cry*]
>
> *Counselor:* It's okay to cry here. Let your feelings out.
>
> *Patient:* [*Still crying*]
>
> *Counselor:* [*Silence*]

Patient: [*Dries her eyes*]

Counselor: What are you feeling right now?

Patient: Just about how complicated my life is. My son's father is in jail—he was abusive toward our son. But my boyfriend is wonderful, and we want to keep it. We have started a new life together, and we want a child together.

Counselor: It sounds like part of you wants to continue the pregnancy. What else is going on for you?

The counselor approached the patient's feelings without assuming the meaning of the patient's tears. It would be understandable to assume that tears upon disclosure of positive results means disappointment, but wait and see what it means to your patient. Sometimes talking about feelings reveals the patient's intentions with regard to this pregnancy. Other times, the patient is just *feeling*—she hasn't yet come to a decision. You can help her to start thinking about her options, even though you won't require that she reach a conclusion.

Exercise 8.6

In your counseling journal, write down each of the following statements made by counselors A, B, C, and D. Think about what each of the statements allows and what each one disallows. Complete this for each of the four statements before reading the discussions that follow.

Counselor A: Do you want to keep the baby or not?

Counselor B: Which option are you going to choose?

Counselor C: What do you think you want to do?

Counselor D: What thoughts do you have about what you might do?

Let's evaluate each of the four counselor responses:

Counselor A: Do you want to keep the baby or not?

What it allows: It doesn't allow much that is positive.

What it disallows: This type of closed-ended question keeps the conversation brief and limits the topics of conversation open to the patient. It disallows a consideration of the full range of pregnancy options. It frames the decision as binary (meaning *two* possible options), which is probably received by most patients as having a choice between parenting and abortion. Adoption is not acknowledged. It also assumes that the patient considers the pregnancy to be a "baby" before listening for the words that the patient uses to describe her pregnancy. By using the verb *keep*, this counselor communicates a judgment that keeping the baby is the preferred or more moral decision. Her word choice implies that abortion is "getting rid of it" and adoption is "giving it away" (see box 8.2).

Box 8.2.   Talking about Parenting

"Continuing the pregnancy and parenting" instead of *"keeping the baby"*

Counselor B: Which option are you going to choose?

What it allows: This is a direct question and implies that the patient has some freedom of choice and that there is more than one option.

What it disallows: The phrasing isn't the best for creating a contemplative space in which to think about options and weigh pros and cons. It sounds like the counselor wants a quick, clear answer from the patient so that she can direct the patient to the right information. For patients whose lives are a bit more complicated and may not feel like they have much of a *choice*, this phrasing can minimize the emotional turmoil and angst that surrounds some pregnancy decisions.

Counselor C: What do you think you want to do?

What it allows: This is an open-ended question that creates a space for the patient to express what she is thinking. If the counselor delivers this question using a gentle, supportive tone of voice, it is likely that the patient will hear the counselor's compassion and desire to help.

What it disallows: The use of the word *want* can be incongruent for some patients who feel that they really don't want any option; none of them seems like a good solution. A lot of women who feel really sure that abortion is the best decision for them still don't *want* to have an abortion; this subtle distinction can communicate that you don't understand your patient's dilemma.

Counselor D: What thoughts do you have about what you might do?

What it allows: This is an open-ended question that creates a space for the patient to express her thoughts. The phrasing communicates the least bias and judgment.

What it disallows: Very little. By guiding the patient to her thoughts, it could direct the conversation away from feelings, but this would be temporary. On the other hand, you could start by asking "What *feelings* do you have about what you might do?" But I find it easier to start with thoughts unless the patient brings up her feelings first. Case example 8.3 continues our analysis of the phrasing used by counselor D.

Case Example 8.3

Counselor: What are you feeling right now?

Patient: [*Starts crying*]

Counselor: It's okay to cry here. Let your feelings out.

Patient: [*Still crying*]

Counselor: [*Silence*]

Patient: [*Sniffles and reaches for a tissue*]

Counselor: What's going on inside?

Patient: I don't even know. I guess I'm in shock.

Counselor: It's okay to not know. I'm here to help you sort through what you're thinking and feeling. Before you came today for your test, what did you think your results might be?

Patient: I thought it might be positive.

Counselor: What were you hoping that your results might be?

Patient: I was hoping that it would be negative.

Counselor: I'm sorry that you didn't get the news that you wanted. At this moment, I can imagine that it's hard for you to picture how you'll find your way through this.

Patient: That's how I feel.

Counselor: Without making any decisions, let's take a moment to think about things. What thoughts do you have about what you might do?

The phrasing of the counselor's last statement is carefully chosen. It initiates the discussion with what the patient is *thinking* and keeps it separate, for the time being, from what she is *feeling*. Sometimes this isn't possible because the patient may lead with her feelings—what her heart wants to do. That's fine; just keep track of whether she is talking about her *head* or her *heart* in a way similar to our work in chapter 6. The use of the word *might* by counselor D is deliberate and meant to imply possibility, not reality. It does not require the patient to commit to any particular option and makes clear that the counselor does not have an agenda; the decision will be made by the patient.

After Disclosing Results

After giving results, the most important thing to do is create a space where the patient can express her feelings and ask questions. Some are hoping for a positive result and know that they want to continue the pregnancy and parent. In those cases, you can focus on determining what help, if any, patients need in finding prenatal care, enrolling in lower-cost food programs, housing, and child care, or obtaining counseling for any psychosocial issues. You'll need to investigate the resources available in your community and refer to those organizations that are culturally and linguistically competent in working with your patient. Some patients will be sure that they want to have an abortion. They may indicate this indirectly; many women seeking abortion care are afraid to use the word *abortion* for fear of stigma and judgment within the health-care system. You can demonstrate your lack of judgment and your openness to abortion by modeling direct communication:

Counselor: What thoughts do you have about what you might do?

Patient: I can't keep it.

Counselor: Are you thinking about abortion as an option for you?

Patient: [Hesitates] Yes.

Counselor: Part of my job here is to help women who want an abortion get all the information that they need to feel more confident and comfortable. I'm happy to help you with that.

Patient: Thank you for saying that. I've been afraid of what people might say if I asked about abortion.

Counselor: That's a very common fear that women have. At this clinic you can ask about anything. There's no judgment here.

Case Example 8.4

Counselor: What thoughts do you have about what you might do?

Patient: I don't want to keep it.

Counselor: So you're thinking that now isn't the right time to continue a pregnancy and become a parent?

Patient: There's no way!

Counselor: That's completely fine. You have two other options to think about. Let's talk about abortion first. What are your thoughts about abortion?

Patient: I've heard that they cut the baby out with a knife, and then you can't get pregnant again. I don't want that to happen to me!

Counselor: Actually, the way that they do the abortion is completely different from that. In fact, no one ever uses a knife in an abortion—there's no cutting at all. And having an abortion won't take away your ability to get pregnant. You now know that you're fertile, and your job from now on will be deciding *when* you want to get pregnant, not *if.* Why don't I take a minute to explain abortion; it might help you in making up your mind about what to do.

This counselor did a good job of clarifying the meaning of the patient's statements so that they were on the same page. She also validated the patient's desire not to continue the pregnancy and parent. You can always return to options that the patient has eliminated if she begins to feel stuck. Here's another example of seeking understanding of the patient's desires and validating her responses:

Counselor: What thoughts do you have about what you might do?

Patient: I don't want to have an abortion. I'm against it.

Counselor: So you're thinking about continuing the pregnancy?

Patient: I'm definitely not going to have an abortion. But after that, I'm not sure.

Counselor: That's completely fine. You have two other options—continuing the pregnancy and parenting or placing the baby for adoption. There are a lot of different adoption options. Let's talk about parenting first. What are your thoughts about parenting?

I often lead with parenting. This communicates that I have no bias against the patient parenting the baby no matter her age, socioeconomic status, or the number of children she already has. This is an essential component of the counselor's approach. Keep in mind that many women and girls have experienced negative judgment surrounding their own or their peers' pregnancy decisions. Because you do not have a personal investment in the outcome of her decision nor do you know what option would be best for her, you are able to present all options in an unbiased, nonjudgmental way. In pregnancy options counseling, we leave our presumption at the door.

Fortunately, the pro-choice adoption movement is gaining more visibility within the family planning and abortion community. We have more opportunities to learn about pro-choice adoption services and feel more confident in our referrals. We can learn more about the adoption experience from birth mothers and adult adopted persons. Two organizations are essential resources for counselors in their education about adoption:

- Backline is a free, confidential talk line where women and men can call to discuss abortion, adoption, and parenting both before and after making a decision. Backline offers trainings for staff on pregnancy options counseling, abortion and adoption counseling, and post-pregnancy support (http://yourbackline.org/).
- The Adoption Access Network (AAN) is a network of adoption agencies in the United States that are pro-choice, woman-centered, support diversity in adoptive families, and work in partnership with abortion providers and family planning clinics. AAN trains staff to become adoption specialists (http://www.adoptionaccessnetwork.org/).

Let's look at an example of how to introduce adoption. This is usually the hardest option for counselors to discuss. This is because we know the least about it. In addition, many health care providers have more negative judgment about adoption than abortion! The problem stems from a lack of information about adoption and the prominence of anti-abortion adoption agencies. We assume that people who support adoption are anti-abortion and see adoption as the moral choice and abortion as the immoral one. The language that we use when talking about adoption has undergone an important transformation to decrease stigma and shame (see box 8.3).

Box 8.3.   Talking about Adoption

"Placing the baby for adoption" instead of *"giving the baby up for adoption"*

Case Example 8.5

Counselor: What thoughts do you have about what you might do?

Patient: I don't want to have an abortion. I'm against it.

Counselor: That's completely fine. You have two other options to think about. Let's talk about parenting first. What are your thoughts about that?

Patient: There's no way that I can have this baby! I'm only sixteen. I need to finish high school and I always planned to go to college. I can't do this!

Counselor: What have you thought about adoption?

Patient: I could never do that. I could never give my baby away.

Counselor: You know, a lot of people say the exact same thing. You're not alone! It's true that adoption may not be for you, but adoption has changed a lot. Modern adoption is a whole new thing. Even though *you* might never do adoption, I like to give girls the information just in case they have a friend who is in a similar circumstance—then you'll be able to tell her what you've learned.

Patient: Okay.

Counselor: Today, girls who decide to place their babies for adoption have a lot more control and are treated a whole lot better. The new way to do adoption is called *open adoption*. That means that you—the birth mother—are treated with respect. You get to choose the family that adopts your baby. You have the right for the baby to know that you are the birth mother. You can even have contact with the baby after the adoption. You and the adoptive family that you choose will make those plans together. Sometimes, girls don't want to see the baby for a while, but when they feel stronger, they want to be able to write letters. Sometimes birth mothers even go and visit. But all of that is up to you and the adoptive family. The arrangements that you make also can change over time so that you can decide how you are feeling as you and the child grow older.

Patient: Wow, I had no idea.

Counselor: Most people don't know, so you're not alone. I like to tell everyone about open adoption; you never know when someone might need the information.

Patient: I think I want to learn more about that.

Counselor: Here's some information on open adoption and the agencies that we like best. The first thing you can do is make a phone call to the agency. There's no pressure; it's okay to explore the idea of adoption even if you change your mind later. You need to get as much information as possible so that you can make the best decision.

Patient: Thank you.

Counselor: You're welcome. Before you go, I want to ask you about your support system. Who else knows that you're pregnant?

At this point, the counselor and patient have found an option that appeals to the patient, at least at this moment. Some readers may be worried about this patient's opinion about abortion. Ask yourself, "Is that because I think it would be better for her to have an abortion?" "Is that because I don't think she'll go through with an adoption?" It would be appropriate for this counselor to check in with the patient and seek understanding of her beliefs about abortion, just in case she was exposed to medical misinformation. She may have eliminated abortion as an option based on fear of how the procedure is performed or its impact on her fertility. You don't have to feel like you've shut the door on talking about other options.

Counselor: I'd also like to check in with you on your feelings about abortion and give you some information in case you have a friend in a similar situation. What do you know about abortion?

Always let the patient know that changing her mind is normal and that you'll be there if she wants to come back and get more information. You can tell her that you want to be sure she has accurate information on her options in case she needs to help someone else in a similar situation. Most clinics have a handout that describes all three options. Patients who initially rejected an option may take the opportunity to read about it later, so be sure that your handouts are accurate and up-to-date. Ask patients to describe their impressions of your handouts; revise them based on their feedback. Too often we use the same handouts for years, not noticing that our language is antiquated or bothering to check whether phone numbers have changed or been disconnected.

When talking about abortion, it is important to emphasize the safety of abortion, the pain control methods that are available at each clinic, and how abortion will not make the patient infertile. It is also important to date her pregnancy so that she knows whether she is eligible for a medication (pill) abortion and at what date she'll move from a one-day (first-trimester) abortion to a two-day (second-trimester) abortion. These guidelines are not hard and fast and may vary across clinics, so you'll need to do your research. Call the abortion clinics in your area to get the following information:

- What is the gestational limit of the clinic?
- What is the cost of abortion services? Does the clinic accept insurance?
- To what gestational duration can the patient have a one-day abortion?
- To what gestational duration can the patient have a medication abortion?
- Are patients referred to another clinic if they have a history of caesarean delivery? What about obesity, asthma, anemia, or other medical issues?
- What options for analgesia and anesthesia does the clinic offer? Do these have an additional cost?
- Do patients need to fast prior to their appointment? Do they need an escort home?
- Does the clinic offer contraception? Which methods are available? What is the cost?

Patients may also have concerns about how the abortion is performed and may have acquired medical misinformation about abortion and fertility. See chapter 6 for a discussion of medical misinformation as a source of decision ambivalence and for a list of resources, books, and handouts to assist patients in making a decision.

FINAL THOUGHTS

Understanding why women have abortions, more than one abortion, or abortions in the second trimester is an important step to developing and maintaining compassion for the patients in your care. Data from many studies about pregnancy incidence are available to help the reader better understand these issues within a woman's life context. We know that women's reasons for having abortions are grounded in their sense of responsibility for the children that they already have and the realization that aspects of their current life situation would negatively affect their ability to care for a child (Finer et al. 2005). This directly counters the claim that abortion decisions are made because women are selfish or irresponsible. Studies seeking to understand why women have more than one abortion instead direct our focus to the factors that contribute to unintended or mistimed pregnancies. Focusing on repeat abortion instead of pregnancy merely serves to increase the stigma of abortion with no mention of the alternative of "repeat child bearing" or the role of men in fertility control (Jones et al. 2006). Women who present for abortion in the second trimester have faced barriers on their journey to accessing care (Drey et al. 2006). Seeking services for later abortion becomes a challenge in the presence of even one of these factors, let alone a conglomeration of multiple hurdles. An accurate understanding of the elements of women's lives that contribute to later abortion is uncommon within the general population, but is essential to the counselor's role as guardian of truth and enemy of stigma.

Similar caveats hold before passing judgment on women who have multiple children or children during their teenage years. Readers have been encouraged to consult the work of Arline T. Geronimus and Kristin Luker to become more enlightened on the complexities of the issue of teenage pregnancy and parenting. Wendy Luttrell's (2003) book *Pregnant Bodies, Fertile Minds* also contributes to our understanding of the experience of teenage parenthood for girls of color. Continuing the pregnancy and parenting is also a politicized issue for adult women. Many aspects of pregnancy, childbirth, and motherhood have been increasingly framed as medically and psychologically hazardous to women (Lee 2003). At the same time parenthood, specifically motherhood, is idealized within our society such that its difficulties and burdens are minimized. A closer glance reveals that this idealization is superficial and insincere. The right to parent has become an issue of economic justice. Just as no woman should be forced to carry a pregnancy to term, policies must change so that no woman is forced to have an abortion because she cannot financially support a baby.

Work in the service of others—whether in the personal or professional realm—starts from a journey within. As you become more confident using the skills that you have learned in this book, reflect upon how you have changed as a person in other aspects of your life. Serenity, deliberateness, humility, and equanimity will increase when you dedicate time and effort to your own growth, development, and change. Every investment in yourself augments your ability to help your patients. Living the principles of this book will help you find a different way of caring for others—one that does not demand the sacrifice of your own sanity and a depletion of your energy. Taking a step back and allowing the patient to lead, to take responsibility for her decisions, and to plan for how she will cope and move forward is the key to your liberation as a counselor and your ability to free others to find their true desires.

Bibliography

Addison, Richard B. 1989. "Grounded Interpretive Research: An Investigation of Physician Socialization." In *Entering the Circle: Hermeneutic Investigation in Psychology*, edited by Martin J. Packer and Richard B. Addison, 39–57. Albany: State University of New York Press.

Adler, Nancy E., Henry P. David, Brenda N. Major, Susan H. Roth, Nancy F. Russo, and Gail E. Wyatt. 1990. "Psychological Responses after Abortion." *Science* 248: 41–44.

———. 1992. "Psychological Factors in Abortion: A Review." *American Psychologist* 47, no. 10 (October): 1194–1204.

American Psychological Association Task Force on Mental Health and Abortion. 2008. *Report of the APA Task Force on Mental Health and Abortion*. Washington, DC: Author. Retrieved from http://www.apa.org/pi/wpo/mental-health-abortion report.pdf.

Appelbaum, Paul S., and Thomas Grisso. 1988. "Assessing Patients' Capacities to Consent to Treatment." *New England Journal of Medicine* 319, no. 25 (December): 1635–38.

Baker, Anne. 1995. *Abortion and Options Counseling: A Comprehensive Reference*. Granite City, IL: Hope Clinic for Women.

———. "Coping Well after an Abortion." Hope Clinic for Women, http://hopeclinic .com/.

Baker, Anne, and Terry Beresford. 2008. "Informed Consent, Patient Education, and Counseling." In *Management of Unintended and Abnormal Pregnancy: Comprehensive Abortion Care*, edited by Maureen Paul, E. Steve Lichtenberg, Lynn Borgatta, David A. Grimes, Phillip G. Stubblefield, and Mitchell. D. Creinin, 48–62. Oxford: Blackwell.

Baker, Anne, and Annie Clark. "Spiritual Comfort: Before and after an Abortion." Hope Clinic for Women, http://hopeclinic.com/.

Baltes, Paul B., and Ursula M. Staudinger. 2000. "Wisdom: A Metaheuristic (Pragmatic) to Orchestrate Mind and Virtue toward Excellence." *American Psychologist* 55, no. 1: 122–36.

Berg, Jessica W., Paul S. Appelbaum, Charles W. Lidz, and Lisa S. Parker. 2001. *Informed Consent: Legal Theory and Clinical Practice*, 2nd ed. New York: Oxford University Press.

Cattaneo, Lauren Bennett, and Aliya R. Chapman. 2010. "The Process of Empowerment: A Model for Use in Research and Practice." *American Psychologist* 65, no.7 (October): 646–59.

Cozzarelli, Catherine, and Brenda Major. 1994. "The Effects of Anti-abortion Demonstrators and Pro-choice Escorts on Women's Psychological Responses to Abortion." *Journal of Social and Clinical Psychology* 13, no. 4: 404–27.

Cozzarelli, Catherine, Brenda Major, Angela Karrasch, and Kathleen Fuegen. 2000. "Women's Experiences of and Reactions to Antiabortion Picketing." *Basic and Applied Social Psychology* 22, no. 4: 265–75.

Cozzarelli, Catherine, Nebi Sumer, and Brenda Major. 1998. "Mental Models of Attachment and Coping with Abortion." *Journal of Personality and Social Psychology* 74, no. 2: 453–67.

Crosby, Maggie C., and Abigail English. 1991. "Mandatory Parental Involvement/ Judicial Bypass Laws: Do They Promote Adolescents' Health?" *Journal of Adolescent Health* 12, no. 2: 143–47.

De Puy, Candace, and Dana Dovitch. 1997. *The Healing Choice: Your Guide to Emotional Recovery after an Abortion*. New York: Fireside.

Drey, Eleanor A., Diana G. Foster, Rebecca A. Jackson, Susan J. Lee, Lilia H. Cardenas, and Philip D. Darney. 2006. "Risk Factors Associated with Presenting for Abortion in the Second Trimester." *Obstetrics and Gynecology* 107, no. 1: 128–35.

Ellenberger, Henri F. 1958. "A Clinical Introduction to Psychiatric Phenomenology and Existential Analysis." In *Existence*, edited by Rollo May, Ernest Angel, and Henri F. Ellenberger, 92–124. New York: Basic Books.

Ellertson, Charlotte. 1997. "Mandatory Parental Involvement in Minors' Abortions: Effects of the Laws in Minnesota, Missouri, and Indiana." *American Journal of Public Health* 87, no. 8: 1367–74.

Festinger, Leon. 1957. *A Theory of Cognitive Dissonance*. Evanston, IL: Row, Peterson.

Finer, Lawrence B., Lori F. Frohwirth, Lindsay A. Dauphinee, Susheela Singh, and Ann M. Moore. 2005. "Reasons U.S. Women Have Abortions: Quantitative and Qualitative Perspectives." *Perspectives on Sexual and Reproductive Health* 37, no. 3: 110–18.

Finer, Lawrence B., and Stanley K. Henshaw. 2006. "Disparities in Rates of Unintended Pregnancy in the United States, 1994 and 2001." *Perspectives on Sexual and Reproductive Health* 39: 90–95.

Fischer, Constance T., ed. 2006. *Qualitative Research Methods for Psychologists: Introduction through Empirical Studies*. San Diego: Academic Press.

Fischer, Constance T., and Frederick J. Wertz. 1979. "Empirical Phenomenological Analyses of Being Criminally Victimized." In Vol. 3 of *Duquesne Studies in*

Phenomenological Psychology, edited by Amadeo Giorgi, Richard Knowles, and David L. Smith, 135–58. Pittsburgh: Duquesne University Press.

Geronimus, Arline T. 2003. "Damned If You Do: Culture, Identity, Privilege and Teenage Childbearing in the United States." *Social Science and Medicine* 57: 881–93.

Gilligan, Carol. 1982. *In a Different Voice: Psychological Theory and Women's Development*. Cambridge: Harvard University Press.

Giorgi, Amadeo. 1970. *Psychology as a Human Science: A Phenomenologically Based Approach*. New York: Harper & Row.

Gold, Rachel Benson, and Elizabeth Nash. 2007. "State Abortion Counseling Policies and the Fundamental Principles of Informed Consent." *Guttmacher Policy Review* 10, no. 4 (Fall): 6–13. Also available online at http://www.guttmacher.org/pubs /gpr/10/4/gpr100406.html.

Gould, Heather, Alissa Perrucci, Rana Barar, and Diana Foster. 2011. "Review of Abortion Patient Information, Education and Emotional Practices in Clinics across the United States." Poster presented at the Thirty-Fifth National Abortion Federation Conference, Chicago.

Grisso, Thomas, and Paul S. Appelbaum. 1995. "Comparison of Standards for Assessing Patients' Capacities to Make Treatment Decisions." *American Journal of Psychiatry* 152: 1033–37.

Grisso, Thomas, Paul S. Appelbaum, and Carolyn Hill-Fotouhi. 1997. "The Mac-CAT-T: A Clinical Tool to Assess Patients' Capacities to Make Treatment Decisions." *Psychiatric Services* 48, no. 11: 1415–19.

Grisso, Thomas, Paul S. Appelbaum, Edward P. Mulvey, and Kenneth Fletcher. 1995. "The MacArthur Treatment Competence Study II." *Law and Human Behavior* 19, no. 2: 127–48.

Hatcher, Robert A., James Trussell, Anita L. Nelson, Willard Cates Jr., Felicia H. Stewart, and Deboral Kowal. 2007. *Contraceptive Technology*, 19th rev. ed. New York: Contraceptive Technology Communications.

Henshaw, Stanley K., and Kathryn Kost. 1992. "Parental Involvement in Minors' Abortion Decisions." *Family Planning Perspectives* 24, no. 5: 196–207, 213.

Johnston, Margaret R. *The Pregnancy Options Workbook*. 1998. Binghamton, NY: Ferre Institute. Also available online at http://www.pregnancyoptions.info/preg nant.htm.

Johnston, Margaret R., and Terry Sallas Merritt. 2008. *A Guide to Emotional and Spiritual Resolution after an Abortion*. Binghamton, NY: Ferre Institute. Also available online at http://www.pregnancyoptions.info/pregnant.htm.

Jones, Rachel K., Alison Purcell, Susheela Singh, and Lawrence B. Finer. 2005. "Adolescents' Reports of Parental Knowledge Adolescents' Use of Sexual Health Services and Their Reactions to Mandated Parental Notification for Prescription Contraception." *Journal of the American Medical Association* 293, no.3: 340–48.

Jones, Rachel K., Susheela Singh, Lawrence B. Finer, and Lori F. Frohwirth. 2006. "Repeat Abortion in the United States." Guttmacher Institute, Occasional Report no. 29 (November). Available online at http://www.guttmacher.org /pubs/2006/11/21/or29.pdf.

Kimport, Katrina. 2010."(Mis)understanding Abortion Regret." Lecture, University of California, San Francisco, September 8.

Lee, Ellie. 2003. *Abortion, Motherhood, and Mental Health: Medicalizing Reproduction in the United States and Great Britain.* New York: Aldine de Gruyter.

Lee, Susan J., Henry J. Peter Ralston, Eleanor A. Drey, John Colin Partridge, and Mark A. Rosen. 2005. "Fetal Pain: A Systematic Multidisciplinary Review of the Evidence." *Journal of the American Medical Association* 294, no. 8 (August 24–31): 947–54.

Lethbridge, Dona J., and Kathleen M. Hanna. 1997. *Promoting Effective Contraceptive Use.* New York: Springer.

Lewis, Catherine. C. 1981. "How Adolescents Approach Decisions: Changes over Grades Seven to Twelve and Policy Implications." *Child Development* 52: 538–44.

Luker, Kristin. 1995. *Dubious Conceptions: The Politics of Teenage Pregnancy.* Cambridge, MA: Harvard University Press.

Luttrell, Wendy. 2003. *Pregnant Bodies, Fertile Minds: Gender, Race, and the Schooling of Pregnant Teens.* New York: Routledge.

Maguire, Daniel C. 2001. *Sacred Choices: The Right to Contraception and Abortion in Ten World Religions.* Minneapolis, MN: Augsburg Fortress.

Major, Brenda, Mark Appelbaum, Linda Beckman, Mary Ann Dutton, Nancy Felipe Russo, and Carolyn West. 2009. "Abortion and Mental Health: Evaluating the Evidence." *American Psychologist* 64, no. 9 (December): 863–90.

Major, Brenda, and Catherine Cozzarelli. 1992. "Psychosocial Predictors of Adjustment to Abortion." *Journal of Social Issues* 48, no. 3: 121–42.

Major, Brenda, Catherine Cozzarelli, M. Lynne Cooper, Josephine Zubek, Caroline Richards, Michael Wilhite, and Richard H. Gramzow. 2000. "Psychological Responses of Women after First-Trimester Abortion." *Archives of General Psychiatry* 57: 777–84.

Major, Brenda, Catherine Cozzarelli, Anne Marie Sciacchitano, M. Lynne Cooper, Maria Testa, and Pallas M. Mueller. 1990. "Perceived Social Support, Self-Efficacy, and Adjustment to Abortion." *Journal of Personality and Social Psychology* 59, no. 3: 452–63.

Major, Brenda, and Richard H. Gramzow. 1999. "Abortion as Stigma: Cognitive and Emotional Implications of Concealment." *Journal of Personality and Social Psychology* 77, no. 4: 735–45.

Major, Brenda, Caroline Richards, M. Lynne Cooper, Catherine Cozzarelli, and Josephine Zubek. 1998. "Personal Resilience, Cognitive Appraisals, and Coping: An Integrative Model of Adjustment to Abortion." *Journal of Personality and Social Psychology* 74, no. 3: 735–52.

May, Rollo. 1958. "Contributions of Existential Psychotherapy." In *Existence,* edited by Rollo May, Ernst Angel, and Henri F. Ellenberger, 37–91. New York: Basic Books.

Melton, Gary B. 1987. "Legal Regulation of Adolescent Abortion: Unintended Effects." *American Psychologist* 42, no. 1 (January): 79–83.

Melton, Gary B., Gerald P. Koocher, and M. J. Saks, eds. 1983. *Children's Competence to Consent.* New York: Plenum.

Miller, William R., and Gary S. Rose. 2009. "Toward a Theory of Motivational Interviewing." *American Psychologist* 64, no. 6 (September): 527–37.

Mueller, Pallas, and Brenda Major. 1989. "Self-Blame, Self-Efficacy, and Adjustment to Abortion." *Journal of Personality and Social Psychology* 57, no. 6: 1059–68.

Needle, Rachel, and Lenore Walker. 2008. *Abortion Counseling: A Clinician's Guide to Psychology, Legislation, Politics, and Competency.* New York: Springer.

Paul, Maureen E., Steve Lichtenberg, Lynn Borgatta, David A. Grimes, Phillip G. Stubblefield, and Mitchell D. Creinin, eds. *Management of Unintended and Abnormal Pregnancy: Comprehensive Abortion Care.* Oxford: Blackwell, 2009.

Perrucci, Alissa. 2006. "The Politics of Fetal Pain." In *Abortion under Attack: Women on the Challenges Facing Choice*, edited by Krista Jacob, 137–42. Emeryville, CA: Seal Press.

Perrucci, Alissa, Sarah Schwartz, and Jennifer Sigafoos. 2007. "The Loss of Confidential Reproductive Health Care Services: Projected Impact on Adolescent Minors." *Policy Briefs and Reports*, California Program on Access to Care (May). Available online at http://www.ucop.edu/cpac/.

Petchesky, Rosalind Pollack. 1998. "Morality and Personhood: A Feminist Perspective." In *The Politics of Women's Bodies: Sexuality, Appearance, and Behavior*, edited by Rose Weitz, 253–69. New York: Oxford University Press.

Pope, Linda M., Nancy E. Adler, and Jeanne M. Tschann. 2001. "Postabortion Psychological Adjustment: Are Minors at Increased Risk?" *Journal of Adolescent Health* 29: 2–11.

Raine, Tina R., Anne Foster-Rosales, Ushma D. Upadhyay, Cherrie B. Boyer, Beth Ann Brown, Abby Sokoloff, and Cynthia C. Harper. 2011."One-Year Contraceptive Continuation and Pregnancy in Adolescent Girls and Women Initiating Hormonal Contraceptives." *Obstetrics and Gynecology* 117, Part 1 (February): 363–71.

Reddy, Diane M., Raymond Fleming, and Carolyne Swain. 2002. "Effect of Mandatory Parental Notification on Adolescent Girls' Use of Sexual Health Care Services." *Journal of the American Medical Association* 288, no. 6: 710–14.

Richardson, Chinue Turner, and Elizabeth Nash. 2006. "Misinformed Consent: The Medical Accuracy of State-Developed Abortion Counseling Materials." *Guttmacher Policy Review* 9, no.4 (Fall): 6–11. Also available online at http://www. guttmacher.org/ pubs/gpr/09/4/gpr090406.html.

Roberts, Dorothy. 1997.*Killing the Black Body: Race, Reproduction, and the Meaning of Liberty.* New York: Vintage.

Rogers, Carl. 1951. *Client-Centered Therapy.* Boston: Houghton Mifflin.

Roth, Loren H., Alan Meisel, and Charles. W. Lidz. 1977. "Tests of Competency to Consent to Treatment." *American Journal of Psychiatry* 134: 279–84.

Runkle, Anna. 1998. *In Good Conscience: A Practical, Emotional, and Spiritual Guide to Deciding Whether to Have an Abortion.* New York: Jossey-Bass.

Russo, Nancy Felipe, and Amy J. Dabul. 1997. "The Relationship of Abortion to Well-Being: Do Race and Religion Make a Difference?" *Professional Psychology: Research and Practice* 28, no. 1: 23–31.

Russo, Nancy F., and Jean E. Denious. 1998. "Why Is Abortion Such a Controversial Issue in the United States?" In *The New Civil War: The Psychology, Culture, and*

Politics of Abortion, edited by Linda J. Beckman and S. Marie Harvey, 25–60. Washington, D.C.: American Psychological Association.

Russo, Nancy F., and Kristin L. Zierk. 1992. "Abortion, Childbearing, and Women's Well-Being." *Professional Psychology: Research and Practice* 23, no. 4: 269–80.

Scherer, David G. 1991. "The Capacities of Minors to Exercise Voluntariness in Medical Treatment Decisions." *Law and Human Behavior* 15, no. 4: 431–49.

Scherer, David G., and N. Dickon Reppucci. 1988. "Adolescents' Capacities to Provide Voluntary Informed Consent." *Law and Human Behavior* 12, no. 2: 123–41.

Shedler, Jonathan. 2010. "The Efficacy of Psychodynamic Psychotherapy." *American Psychologist* 65, no. 2 (February–March): 98–109.

Speroff, Leon, and Philip D. Darney. 2005. *A Clinical Guide for Contraception*, 4th ed. Philadelphia, PA: Lippincott.

Steinberg, Julia R., Davida Becker, and Jillian T. Henderson. 2011. "Does the Outcome of a First Pregnancy Predict Depression, Suicidal Ideation, or Lower Self-Esteem? Data from the National Comorbidity Survey." *American Journal of Orthopsychiatry* 81, no. 2: 193–201.

Steinberg, Julia Renee, and Nancy F. Russo. 2008. "Abortion and Anxiety: What's the Relationship?" *Social Science & Medicine* 67: 238–52.

Steinberg, Laurence, Elizabeth Cauffman, Jennifer Woolard, Sandra Graham, and Marie Banich. 2009. "Are Adolescents Less Mature Than Adults? Minors' Access to Abortion, the Juvenile Death Penalty, and the Alleged APA 'Flip Flop.'" *American Psychologist* 64, no. 7: 583–94.

Teyber, Edward. 1992. *Interpersonal Process in Psychotherapy*, 2nd ed. Pacific Grove, CA: Brooks/Cole.

Torre-Bueno, Ava. 1997. *Peace after Abortion*. San Diego: Pimpernel Press.

Torres, Aida, and Jacqueline Darroch Forrest. 1988. "Why Do Women Have Abortions?" *Family Planning Perspectives* 20, no. 4 (July–August): 169–76.

Trybulski, JoAnn. 2006. "The Long-Term Phenomena of Women's Postabortion Experiences: Reply to the Letter to the Editor." *Western Journal of Nursing Research* 28: 354–56.

Upadhyay, Ushma D., Kate Cockrill, and Lori R. Freedman. 2010. "Informing Abortion Counseling: An Examination of Evidence-Based Practices Used in Emotional Care for Other Stigmatized and Sensitive Health Issues." *Patient Education and Counseling* 81: 415–21.

Walsh, Russell. 2003. "The Methods of Reflexivity." *The Humanistic Psychologist* 31: 332–44.

Weithorn, Lois A., and Susan B. Campbell. 1982. "The Competency of Children and Adolescents to Make Informed Treatment Decisions." *Child Development* 53, no. 6: 1589–98.

Wertz, Frederick J. 2005. "Phenomenological Research Methods for Counseling Psychology." *Journal of Counseling Psychology* 52, no. 2: 167–77.

Index

abortion: and empowerment, xxii-iv;
    existential meaning of, xv-vi; junk
    science and, 14; as a life event,
    xxii, 9, 13; as a moral decision, 8,
    48, 51, 55–56, 76, 79, 99–100, 107;
    psychological response after, 9–13;
    and the value of human life, xxiv;
    and women's personhood, xv, xxiv;
    women's reasons for, 192
Abortion Care Network, xiv, 84
Abortion Conversation Project, xiii-iv
abortion counseling: definition of, xxiv,
    1; components of, 1–7, *3*; patient
    concerns about, 20; purpose of, xxi,
    9
adolescents: coercion and, 162–63;
    informed consent and, 161–62;
    and parenting, 163–65; research on
    abortion and, 10–11, 13; talking to
    parents of, 166–70; voluntariness of
    decisions, 160
adoption: bias against, 121–22; 174;
    case examples of, 139–40, 148–49,
    165, 167, 188, 189–90; informed
    consent and, 155, 159–60; patient
    conflict with, 71, 120, 123, 130;
    patient consideration of, 128–29,
    131, 141; pro-choice, 127, 188–89;
    reframing and, 126–27; talking

about, 72–73, 119, 132, 141, 179;
    184–85, *189*
Adoption Access Network, 127, 189
aftercare, 1, 2, 4–5, 170, *171*
ambivalence, 117–19, 152; approach
    and, 121–22; definition of, 119–21;
    framework and, 122; reframing,
    126–44; seeking understanding of,
    123–26; validating and normalizing,
    122–23
approach, definition of, xxi-ii, 15–17

Backline, 46, 152, 189
Baker, Anne, xiii-xiv, 5, 46, 85
Baxter, Darcy, 76

certainty scale (counseling tool), 124–
    25, 136–37, 145
continuing the pregnancy. *See* adoption;
    parenting
contraception: coercive promotion
    of, 6; health education for, xxiv,
    1–6; men's role in, 52, 80, 84; and
    religion, 80

decision assessment: definition of, 6–8,
    19, 26; case examples of, 21–22, 28;
    steps of, 7, 20–21, *21*; theory behind,
    9, 22

emotional conflict: approach and,
28–29; decision counseling for, *53*;
definition of, 27; reframing, 48–57;
and relationships, 45, 110, 136;
seeking understanding of, 33–47, *37*;
validating and normalizing, 30–33
Exhale, 46, 152

Faith Aloud, 46, 60, 80, 82, 84, 152
fetal pain, 36–39, 44, 46, 126–28
framework, definition of, xxi-ii, 8, *8*

grief, 27, 36, 42, 45, 54, 84, 88, 106
guilt, 44, 46–47, 49, 95, 101, 106–7,
125–6, 128, 138

health education. *See* contraception
hypothetical situations (counseling tool),
132–34, 142–43

informed consent, 172; adolescents and,
see adolescents; definition, 153–54;
components of, *154*, 155–61;
documentation for, 170–72

Johnston, Margaret (Peg). *See*
Pregnancy Options Workbook

killing: definition of, 93; emotional
conflict and, 36–41, 147; spiritual
conflict and, 70, 75, 80, 82–83;
moral conflict and, 87, 89–90,
93–96, 101, 109–111, 135; *see also*
murder

listen-put forward-dwell (counseling
tool), 128–31, *129*

moral conflict: approach and, 90;
challenging case examples of,
104–15; cognitive dissonance and,
89–90, 98; decision counseling for,
98; definition of, 87–88; informed
consent and, 88, 115; reframing,
97–104; seeking understanding of,

93–97; validating and normalizing,
91–92
murder: definition of, 93; moral conflict
and abortion as, 87–90, 93–94, 100–
101, 105, 108–15; *See also* killing

National Abortion Federation, 6
normalization, purposeful, xxii-iv, 76

parenting: case examples of, 137–40,
147–49, 167–69, 188–89; bias
against, 161, 174, 177–78, 192–93;
emotional health and, 9–10; informed
consent and, 159–60, 162; patient
conflict with, 119–23, 130, 134;
patient consideration of, 128–29;
reality testing for, 163–64; talking
about, 71–74, 101–5, 131–33, 141,
184–85, *185*, 188
Peace After Abortion, 84, 151
peer counseling, xxiii
philosophical ground, xv-vi, 63, 115
post-abortion coping: case examples of
planning for, 24, 36; and emotional
health, 13b; planning for, 23–24, 26,
45–46, 84–85; research on, 11–13,
12
Pregnancy Options Workbook, xiv, 45,
151, 164
pregnancy test counseling, 173;
179–92
psychosocial assessment, *7*, 13

reality check (counseling tool), 40, 134
reflecting back (counseling tool), 16, 43,
50, 57, 98, 111, 122, 130, 140–41,
148–49
reframing, introduction to, 7–8, 27–28,
37, 47–48, 50, 53, 55–57
regret: abortion and, 15–16, 27, 30, 87,
89; case examples of, 113, 143–44,
159; reframing, 51–53
Religious Coalition for Reproductive
Choice, 60, 80, 85
Runkle, Anna, 151

selfishness: abortion as, 27, 44, 125, 192; case examples of, 49–50, 54, 69, 78–79, 128, 138; reframing, 50–51, 76, 79

shame, 37, 44, 70, 89, 106, 174–75

six dimensions of pregnancy decision making (counseling tool), 123, *124*, 129, 139, 142

social support, 10–13, *12*, 22–25, 27, 33

spiritual conflict: approach and, 61; decision counseling for, *77*; definition of, 59–60; forgiveness and, 65–66, *65*, *67*; judgment from God and, 82–83; punishment from God and, *70*, 73, 80–82; reframing, 76–85; religion and, 59–63, 80; seeking understanding of, 64–76;

sin and, 66–67, 71, 74–76, 78–79; validating and normalizing, 63–64

stigma, xxi-ii, 182, 187, 192; adoption and, 189, *189*; anti-abortion movement and, 14, 30; research on, 12, *12*; removing, xxii-iii, 8, 16, 20, 53, 57, 85

Taft, Charlotte. *See* Abortion Care Network

teens. *See* adolescents

Torre-Bueno, Ava. *See* Peace After Abortion

Turner, Reverend Rebecca. *See* Faith Aloud

values clarification, 173–79

About the Author

Alissa C. Perrucci, PhD, MPH, is a chief community health program manager at the University of California, San Francisco.